Dr Ante Bilić
liječnik - stomatolog

Ante Bilić
29. 02. 1984

Surgery of
the Salivary Glands

DALE H. RICE, M.D.
Associate Professor and Vice-chief
Head and Neck Surgery
UCLA School of Medicine
and
Chief
Head and Neck Surgery
Veterans Administration
Wadsworth Medical Center
Los Angeles, California

1982
B.C. Decker Inc. • Trenton, New Jersey
The C.V. Mosby Company • Saint Louis • Toronto • London

Publisher: B. C. Decker Inc.
            3 Belmont Circle
            Trenton, NJ 08618

in Canada: 3228 South Service Road
            Burlington, Ontario L7N3H8

U.S.A. and worldwide sales and distribution by:
            The C. V. Mosby Company
            11830 Westline Industrial Drive
            St. Louis, Missouri 63141

in Canada: The C. V. Mosby Company
            120 Melford Drive
            Toronto, Ontario M1B2X5

Surgery of the Salivary Glands   ISBN 0-941158-00-4

Library of Congress catalog card number: 82-072571

Last digit is print number: 10   9   8   7   6   5   4   3   2   1

PREFACE

This book is the result of a professional lifelong interest in the salivary glands and the diseases that affect them. The salivary glands are beset by a greater variety of ills than any other tissue in the body and advances in research are occurring on a daily basis. Therefore, I have no reason to believe this book to be up-to-the-minute, but I have attempted to be as contemporary as possible.

While the book has a clinicopathological orientation, I have included basic anatomic, physiologic, and biochemical data as a necessary background for understanding the various clinical entities discussed. In all chapters I have attempted to be comprehensive but not encyclopedic. The book is intended to be a clinical reference to diseases that affect the salivary glands. The text has been liberally referenced, but I have generally adhered to a policy of citing the original or what I consider to be the best reference when multiple references are available. Where there is a divergence of opinion I have given both sides, usually followed by my personal solution to the problem.

There are many to thank. I had the good fortune of doing my residency at the University of Michigan under the chairmanship of Walter P. Work, M.D. Doctor Work set personal standards of intellectual honesty, clinical acumen, persuit of excellence and compassion every physician would do well to emulate. Further, he attracted a staff of exceptional teachers—names well-known in Otolaryngolygy/Head and Neck Surgery— Roger Boles, M.D., George Gates, M.D. Nels Olsen, M.D., Frank Ritler, M.D., Stanley Coulthard, M.D. Together they created an intellectual environment with an expectation of excellence that encouraged unfettered development.

That experience was further enhanced by having as a friend and teacher from medical school to the present John G. Batsakis, M.D.—a brilliant and tireless repository of information. My early breakfasts with him proved to be the best educational investment per unit of time in my life.

Leonardo de Vinci said, "The student who does not surpass his master has failed his master." For those of us who trained at the University of Michigan during that era, this will be a long and difficult, if even possible, task.

Since completing my residency, I have been at UCLA where Paul Ward, M.D. and Thomas Calcaterra, M.D. have added substantially to my education.

The final person responsible for this book is Margaret Bailey, the world's best secretary, administrator, and right hand.

TO

Walter P. Work, M.D.
and
John G. Batsakis, M.D.

CONTENTS

Chapter One

STRUCTURE AND FUNCTION OF THE SALIVARY GLANDS

ANATOMY

Embryology

The embryology of the salivary glands is incompletely understood. The major salivary glands and the minor glands anterior to the anterior tonsillar pillars are believed to be derived from ectoderm, whereas the remaining glands are derived from endoderm. However, there is no histologic difference between the two areas, and no difference in the tumors that occur there.

Proliferating buds penetrate the surrounding mesenchyme. The buds arborize to a variable degree, finally terminating as acini. The parotid develops first, beginning at about the fourth week of intrauterine life. It begins at the corner of the mouth, but ends opposite the second maxillary molar because of intervening mesodermal proliferation. As the gland arborizes posteriorly, the facial nerve migrates anteriorly through it. Since parotid ductal branching and facial nerve migration occur before the condensation of mesenchyme, the gland and nerve develop an intimate relationship, with major portions of the nerve being completely surrounded by the gland. As the mesenchyme condenses it divides the parotid into small compartments with strong fibrous septa. These septa prevent parotid abscesses from becoming fluctuant. In addition, they are continuous with the enveloping superfical layer of deep cervical fascia, which prevents the development of a surgical plane between the fascia and the parotid. Numerous lymph nodes develop adjacent to and within the parotid, and salivary gland tissue has been found within these nodes.[1] Sebaceous glands also occur within the parotid and are thought to originate from the intercalated and striated ducts.[2] The parotid is largely or exclusively serous.

The submandibular gland begins to develop in the sixth week of intrauterine life. Unlike the parotid it develops as a relatively discrete structure with early condensation of its surrounding mesenchyme. Thus

3

other structures do not occur within the substance of the gland. In particular, lymph nodes lie adjacent to, but not within, it. The submandibular gland acini are seromucous.

The sublingual gland begins to develop in the eighth week and is also a rather discrete structure. It lies lateral to the submandibular duct and medial to the mylohyoid muscle. The sublingual gland is largely mucous. The minor salivary glands begin to form about the twelfth week and are widely scattered throughout the oral cavity except on the alveolar ridges and the anterior hard palate. They may be serous, mucous, or mixed.

Histology

The mature salivary gland unit begins as a serous or mucous acinus (Figure 1–1). Acini empty into an intercalated duct, which in turn leads to a striated duct that empties into an excretory duct. The excretory duct forms the collecting tubes for saliva. Each salivary gland segment has specialized functional and morphologic characteristics.

Acinar cells are highly differentiated cells responsible for the production of mucinous or serous secretions. These cells contain well-developed rough endoplasmic reticulum and Golgi bodies with abundant secretory granules. Parotid acini are predominately or exclusively serous, whereas those of the submandibular gland are of a single type called seromucous.[3] The mucous acini of the sublingual gland resemble those of the submandibular gland. Unmyelinated nerve terminals with numerous synaptic vesicles exist between the acinar cells, indicating autonomic innervation.

ACINUS INTERCALATED STRIATED EXCRETORY
DUCT   DUCT   DUCT

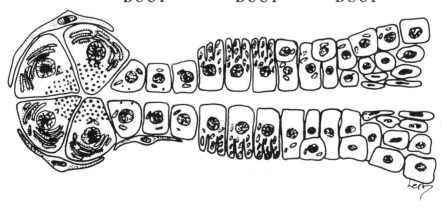

Figure 1–1. Histology of mature salivary unit.

TABLE 1–1   Histogenesis of Salivary Gland Tumors

	Benign	*Malignant*
Intercalated duct reserve cell	Papillary adenoma Pleomorphic adenoma Monomorphic adenomas	Adenoid cystic carcinoma Acinious cell carcinoma
Excretory duct reserve cell	Intraductal papilloma	Squamous cell carcinoma Mucoepidermoid carcinoma Adenocarcinoma
Uncertain	Warthin's tumor Oncocytoma	

The cuboidal cells of the intercalated duct are relatively unspecialized. In contrast, the striated duct cells are well differentiated and show features common to the renal proximal tubule cells. The striated duct cells play an important role in electrolyte and water transportation. The myoepithelial cells were first described in 1898 and are located around the periphery of the acini and the intercalated ducts. They appear to have the ability to contract[4] and thus expel saliva from the acini. They also seem to play a role in transport and basement membrane function.

The basal cells of the intercalated and excretory ducts act as reserve cells for the more differentiated cells of the salivary gland unit. Thus these two cells are not only responsible for normal salivary gland development, but for tumor formation also.[5] It is now generally agreed that salivary gland tumors arise from one of these two cells, and data from both light microscopic and electron microscopic studies support this theory[6] (Table 1–1).

Gross Anatomy

The parotid gland is the largest salivary gland and lies anterior and inferior to the ear (Figure 1–2). It overlies the upper one-fourth of the sternocleidomastoid muscle, and the masseter muscle, while the deep lobe extends medially between the ascending ramus of the mandible and the mastoid process. The deep lobe is merely a medial extension of the parotid gland and is not a true separate lobe, but common usage has designated it as such and that use will be continued here. The gland is enveloped by the superficial layer of the deep cervical fascia, which is continuous with the fibrous septa of the gland itself. At its lower pole, the parotid is separated from the tail of the submandibular gland by a condensation of the fascia, the stylomandibular ligament (quadrangular fascia). The superficial por-

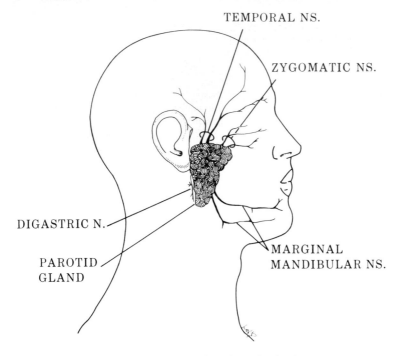

Figure 1–2. Anatomic location of parotid gland.

tion of the gland is subcutaneous. The anterior border overlies the masseter muscle. The parotid (Stenson's) duct, often accompanied by accessory parotid tissue, exits the anterior border, passes anteriorly across the masseter muscle approximately midway between the zygomatic arch and the corner of the mouth, turns medially at the anterior border of the masseter, penetrates the buccinator muscle, and opens into the oral cavity at a level corresponding to the junction of the root and the crown of the maxillary second molar (teeth numbers 2 and 15). The transverse facial artery and vein parallel the duct superiorly. The branches of the facial nerve also exit the gland along the anterior border and radiate across the masseter and the zygomatic arch. The superior border of the gland lies inferior to the zygomatic arch, and from it exits the temporal branch of the facial nerve, the superficial temporal artery and vein, and the auriculotemporal nerve (the latter implicated in gustatory sweating or Frey's syndrome). The medial surface of the gland lies on the masseter or sternocleidomastoid muscles or extends between the mandible and the mastoid process. In the medial portion of the gland (medial to the facial nerve) lie the external carotid artery and the posterior facial vein. The artery divides into the superficial temporal and internal maxillary arteries, and the vein receives the corresponding veins. The deep auricular and transverse facial arteries also arise here. The anteromedial portion of the deep lobe is related to the internal jugular vein, the internal carotid artery, and the styloid process and its muscles. The posterior belly of the digastric muscle borders the deep lobe posteromedially. Anterosuperiorly, the deep lobe abuts the ascending ramus of the mandible and the posterior border of the medial pterygoid muscle. Posteriorly, the deep lobe is adjacent to the mastoid process and the external auditory canal. The blood supply to the gland comes from the vessels traversing it.

The relationship of the parotid gland to the facial nerve is of major importance to the surgeon. Were the nerve not within the gland, parotidectomy would be a simple procedure. The facial nerve exits the temporal bone via the stylomastoid foramen typically crossing the posterolateral aspect of the styloid process and quickly enters the parotid. Prior to entering the parotid, the facial nerve gives off posterior auricular, posterior belly of digastric, and stylohyoid branches, but these are of little consequence in parotid disease. The first major division of the nerve (pes anserinus) occurs approximately 1.3 cm from the stylomastoid foramen into the temperofacial and cervicofacial branches. Throughout its intraglandular course, the facial nerve is intimately interwoven with parotid tissue. The temperofacial and cervicofacial branches may pass through the parotid without anastomosis, but more commonly these divisions and their branches have multiple anastomoses to form the parotid plexus. The anastomotic pattern is quite variable and the marginal mandibular and cervical branches usually do not participate. That means the lower branches are typically single, while the upper branches are functionally multiple. The designation of branches as temporal, zygomatic, buccal, marginal mandibular, and cervical do not describe true individual branches, but rather areas of distribution. Anatomic studies have demonstrated eight major branching patterns[7] (Figure 1–3).

The submandibular gland occupies most of the submandibular triangle. The inferior surface lies adjacent to the anterior and posterior bellies of the digastric muscle. The superficial surface is crossed by the anterior facial vein and, in a small percentage of cases, the marginal mandibular branch of the facial nerve. In the anatomic position, 80 per cent of marginal mandibular branches pass no lower than the lower border of the mandible. In the surgical position, with the head turned and extended, the marginal mandibular branch is usually pulled below the mandible. A variable number of lymph nodes also lie along the superior superficial aspect of the gland. The facial artery passes across the upper surface of the gland before rounding the lower border of the mandible. Anteriorly the gland lies directly on the mylohyoid muscle. Deep to the gland lie the lingual and hypoglossal nerves, and the hyoglossus muscle. The lingual nerve gives a

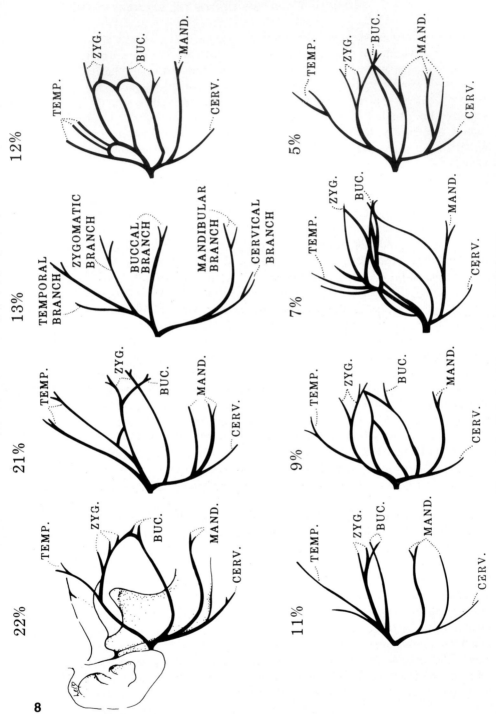

Figure 1-3. Major branching patterns of facial nerve.

8

branch to the gland. The submandibular (Wharton's) duct, with a deep portion of the gland, passes anteriorly between the mandible and the hyoglossus and genioglossus muscles. It is crossed first laterally and then medially by the lingual nerve as it passes anteriorly. Finally the duct passes medial to the sublingual gland and empties into the floor of the mouth lateral to the frenulum.

The sublingual gland lies below the mucosa of the floor of the mouth anteriorly, superficial to the mylohyoid muscle. It is bounded laterally by the mandible and medially by the styloglossus, hyoglossus, and genioglossus muscles. The hypoglossal and lingual nerves pass between the sublingual gland and the genioglossus muscle to enter the tongue. The sublingual ducts are approximately 12 in number and either empty directly into the floor of the mouth or into the submandibular duct.

Operative Anatomy for Parotidectomy

The patient is first placed under endotracheal general anesthesia. When appropriate, hypotensive techniques substantially decrease intraoperative bleeding, which can be particularly bothersome when it obscures identification of the main trunk of the facial nerve. Another useful method of decreasing intraoperative bleeding is to mix 3 cc of 1:1000 epinepherine with 30 cc of sterile saline and to inject 5 to 10 cc of this mixture into the incision and operative site between the tragus and the posterior belly of the digastric muscle. The patient is next positioned, with the head turned to the side opposite the lesion and extended by placing a towel roll under the ipsilateral shoulder. The entire hemiface and neck is washed with povidone-iodine. Draping is performed with towels in a way that permits the entire hemiface to be visible. A transparent plastic self-sticking drape is then applied to the face anterior to the line of the incision to keep the entire hemiface visible without interfering with the incision or the closure. The incision is a triple modified Blair incision. The original Blair incision began superiorly by paralleling the last centimeter of the zygomatic arch, then turned sharply inferiorly, passed anterior to the ear, and continued into the neck along the anterior border of the sternocleidomastoid muscle. Currently, the part parelleling the zygomatic arch has been eliminated. The incision begins superiorly, immediately anterior to the helical rim, passes between it and the tragus, continues inferiorly on the posterior surface of the tragus, curves anteriorly between the tragus and the lobule, curves posteriorly under the lobule to the mastoid process, then curves gently inferiorly to pass into the neck in a natural wrinkle if one is present in an appropriate location (Figure 1–4). Careful closure of this incision will

ERRATUM

0.3 cc 1:1000

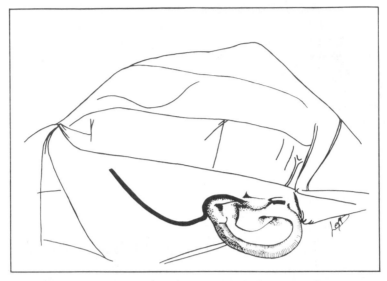

DRAPING SO THAT ENTIRE HEMIFACE IS VISIBLE
INCISION-PART ON POSTERIOR SURFACE OF
TRAGUS CANNOT BE SEEN

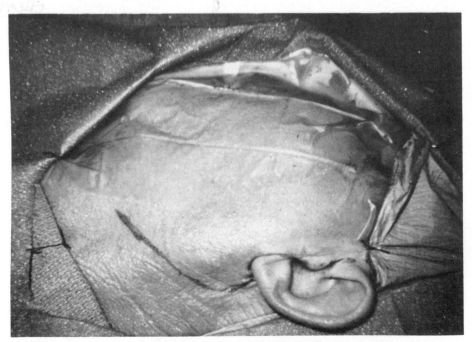

Figure 1–4. (Legend on page 12)

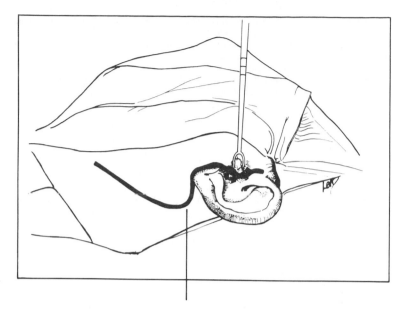

INCISION WITH PART CARRIED ON
POSTERIOR SURFACE OF TRAGUS

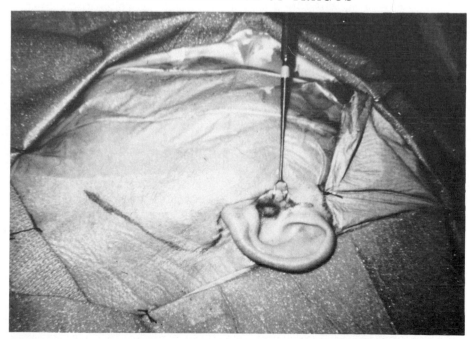

Figure 1–4 (pp. 10 and 11). Photographs and corresponding line drawings showing draping for parotidectomy and the incision used. For most parotidectomies I prefer the standard doubly modified Blair incision with a third modification. The latter modification involves carrying the pre-auricular incision behind the tragus as many do for rhytidectomy. This serves to break up the long vertical pre-auricular incision for better camouflage. The curve of the incision posterior and inferior to the lobule is a gentle one that then continues into a convenient neck wrinkle at approximately hyoid level or slightly higher. The original Blair incision had an anterior extension parallel to the zygomatic arch and came to a sharp point over the mastoid tip.

I prefer to use a plastic transparent drape over the entire hemiface so that facial nerve activity can be easily assessed. I place the drape anterior to the incision so that it does not interfere with the incision or the closure.

The table should be positioned with the head slightly elevated to decrease venous and capillary oozing. The injection of a dilute epinephrine solution into the incision line and the area of the main trunk of the facial nerve and hypotensive anesthesia are ancillary techniques that will also decrease troublesome bleeding during identification of the main trunk of the facial nerve.

yield an almost imperceptible scar. The flap is elevated sharply to the anterior border of the gland to expose the operative field.

"The structures that surround the gland command more attention than details of the gland itself."[8] The structure that commands the most attention is the facial nerve. The only constant location of the facial nerve is at the stylomastoid foramen, posterior and lateral to the base of the styloid process. In general, then, this is the preferred location to attempt identification of the nerve. At a point approximately two-thirds of the distance from the angle of the mandible to the temperomandibular joint, the main trunk divides into the temperofacial and the cervicofacial branches. More distal branching is highly variable (q.v.), and peripheral branches often are not in the same parasagittal plane, with the superior branches usually more superficial than the inferior branches. The nerve is surrounded by a thin sleeve of connective tissue allowing separation of the gland from the nerve.

Mobilization of the posterior surface of the gland is the key to rapid identification of the nerve. The gland is first separated from the cartilaginous and bony ear canal by blunt dissection following the tragal perichondrium until the styloid process can be readily palpated (Figure 1–5). Next the gland is separated from the anterior border of the sternocleidomastoid muscle, and this separation requires division of the anterior branch of the great auricular nerve. If resection of part of the facial nerve is anticipated, the great auricular nerve can be dissected out and saved for use as a graft in repairing the facial nerve following resection of the tumor. The gland is reflected forward until the posterior belly of the digastric can be seen. The main trunk now lies within a triangle formed by the tragal cartilage (posterior), the posterior belly of the digastric, and the styloid process (Figure 1–6). The dissection should thus continue toward the styloid process from the tragal pointer and the digastric. The main trunk is usually greater than 1 cm deep to and slightly inferior to the tragal

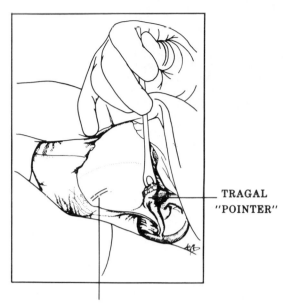

TRAGAL
"POINTER"

GREAT AURICULAR NERVE

PHOTOGRAPH SHOWING EXPOSURE OF GLAND
AND TRAGAL "POINTER"

Figure 1–5. Photograph and corresponding line drawing showing identification of the "tragal pointer." There are at least two methods of identifying the main trunk of the facial nerve, as mentioned in the text. For the purposes of resident teaching I prefer to dissect out in turn the tragal pointer and the posterior belly of the digastric muscle. At this point the styloid process can be palpated between them. The facial nerve passes over the posterior-inferior aspect of the styloid process. Careful blunt spreading in this area allows rapid identification of the main trunk with little chance of damage to the nerve.

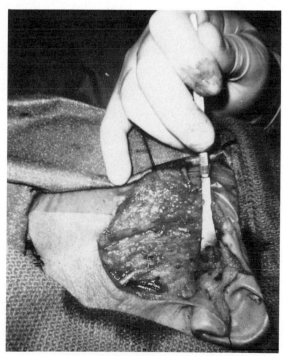

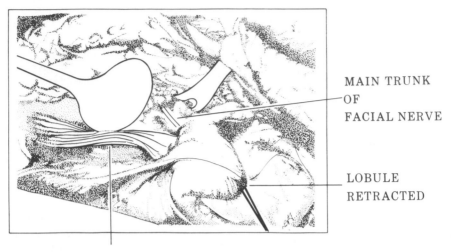

MAIN TRUNK
OF
FACIAL NERVE

LOBULE
RETRACTED

DIGASTRIC MUSCLE

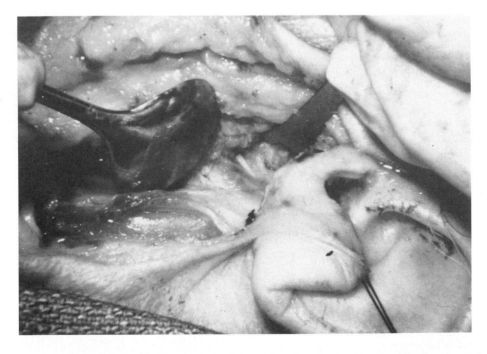

Figure 1–6. Photograph and corresponding line drawing showing identification of the main trunk of the facial nerve and its relationship to the "tragal pointer" and the posterior belly of the digastric muscle. Once the main trunk of the facial nerve is identified the operation is merely a branch-by-branch dissection of the facial nerve. The safest course of action is to first follow the branch farthest from the tumor. Upon completion of this part the parotid will be divided into two portions, one of which

pointer and is surrounded by a small amount of fat—a warning of its proximity. An alternate, but equally satisfactory, technique is to follow the tympanomastoid suture medially. The main trunk of the facial nerve will be found 6 to 8 mm deep to its drop-off point.[9]

In the rare situation in which the main trunk cannot be safely approached, there are six optional approaches. Five of these involve identifying a peripheral branch and following it retrograde to the main trunk. The buccal branch is parallel to and approximately 1 cm inferior to the zygomatic arch and slightly superior to the parotid duct. The marginal mandibular branch can be found by carefully dissecting along the deep surface of the tail of the gland. Eye branches can be identified by careful dissection along the zygomatic arch. The cervical branch can be located by dissecting along the posterior, deep surface of the tail of the gland. Finally the posterior facial vein can be located inferior to the gland and followed superiorly until the cervicofacial branch crosses it superficially. The sixth method involves partial removal of the mastoid process to identify the main trunk prior to its exit from the temporal bone.

Once the main trunk is identified, the operation becomes a branch-by-branch dissection of the nerve. A fine-tipped hemostat (there are special hemostats designed for this purpose) is passed along the lateral surface of the nerve and then raised off it. This is best done in a single motion. The beginning parotid surgeon seems to have an almost uncontrollable urge to make this motion several times. This is unnecessary and adds additional trauma to the nerve. The parotid tissue between the tips is then incised. Each side is clamped with a hemostat to control bleeding and to act as a retractor. At the pes anserinus, the branch leading away from the tumor is followed until it exits the gland. This divides the parotid into two portions, a large portion containing the tumor and a small portion. The latter is easily and rapidly excised. Attention is then directed to the larger portion, which is removed by dissecting out each branch in turn while "rolling" the tissue off the nerve (Figure 1–7).

Contemporary thinking favors total parotidectomy as the basic procedure for all parotid neoplasms regardless of location. The deep lobe is approached, only after removal of the superficial lobe, from below the facial nerve. For deep lobe neoplasms, incision of the stylomandibular ligament and fracture of the styloid process may be necessary. On rare occasions, mandibulotomy may be necessary. A useful maneuver is to place a finger in the oral cavity and manually displace the tumor laterally.

contains the tumor and one of which does not. The parotid is then dissected off the nerve branch-by-branch, moving inferiorly or superiorly until it is completely free of the facial nerve. Thus the gland is "rolled" superiorly or inferiorly while each branch encountered is dissected free.

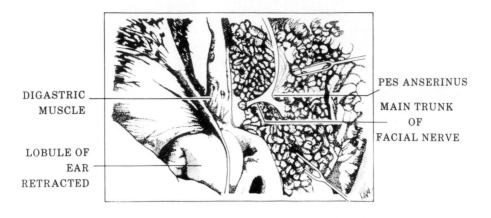

DIGASTRIC
MUSCLE

LOBULE OF
EAR
RETRACTED

PES ANSERINUS

MAIN TRUNK
OF
FACIAL NERVE

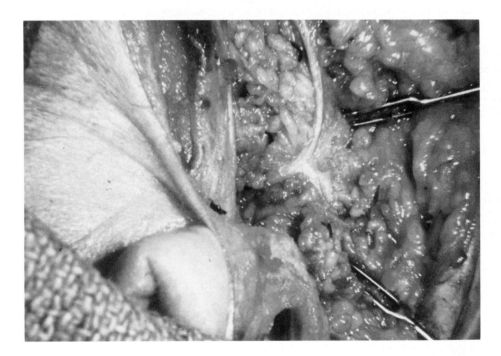

Figure 1–7 Photograph and line drawing showing partially completed parotidectomy with exposure of pes anserinus and cervicofacial branch. Parotid tissue still covers upper branches. At the completion of the parotidectomy it is imperative to ascertain that all branches work. A single stimulation of the main trunk should demonstrate this. This fact should be entered into the operative note. If any branch fails to produce motion, it should be carefully inspected. If it is found to be disrupted, it should be immediately repaired. One surgeon I know routinely photographs the intact facial nerve and its branches immediately prior to closure.

These principles apply whether the tumor is unilobular or dumbbell in shape. The unilobular deep lobe tumor most commonly appears as a submucosal parapharyngeal mass, whereas the dumbbell tumor also shows a mass at the angle of the mandible.

At the termination of the procedure the wound should be thoroughly irrigated in an attempt to wash out any tumor cells that may have spilled. Facial nerve function should be checked immediately prior to skin closure. The branch to any area that does not function should be investigated and repaired if found to be severed. The preferred method of stimulation is with an adjustable square-wave electrical unit. Disposable units appear to act as a small cautery and may cause permanent damage to the nerve.[10] If all branches function properly when stimulated at one-quarter volt at one-thirtieth ampere, the facial nerve will function normally in the recovery room.

Should any branch of the facial nerve be severed inadvertently or deliberately resected, causing a region of the face to be immobile, repair should be performed during the initial operation. Direct repair gives the best results. If only a short segment of nerve has been resected or the nerve inadvertently severed, direct end-to-end anastomosis gives the optimum result. If direct end-to-end anastomosis is not possible, but both ends of the nerve are available, a cable graft should be performed, using such excellent donor nerves as the great auricular and the anterior or lateral femoral cutaneous nerves. It may even be necessary to enter the temporal bone to find the proximal nerve trunk. If, for any reason, the proximal trunk is not available, the best rehabilitation can be obtained with a hypoglossal-facial anastomosis,[11] which usually restores tone and motion, especially to the lower face. Other repairs occasionally used are the spinal accessory-facial and the phrenic-facial anastomoses. Nerve repair can usually be performed with unaided vision using 8-0, 9-0, or 10-0 monofilament silk. There is some controversy concerning the optimal technique of repair. Some investigators favor interfascicular repair.[12] The best results, however, appear to follow closure of the epineurium.[13] Two to seven sutures through the epineurium only appear to give the best results. For small branches, magnifying loupes or the operating microscope may be useful. Placing a material with a contrasting color beneath the nerve ends often facilitates the repair.

Numerous techniques are available for secondary rehabilitation or when the distal facial branches are unavailable. The most popular of these utilize slings of temporalis or masseter muscle to support the corner of the mouth and eyelids. Recently nerve-muscle pedicle techniques have been extended from use in reinnervating the larynx to reinnervating the face.[14] All of these techniques are distinctly inferior to direct nerve repair.

PHYSIOLOGY

Secretory Unit

The secretory unit of the salivary gland is composed of the acini, the intercalated ducts, and the striated ducts. The acinar cells are arranged around a central lumen and have myoepithelial cells interposed between them and the basement membrane peripherally. Serous cells produce a watery secretion containing neutral carbohydrates; mucous cells secrete a viscous solution with mucopolysaccharides; seromucous cells secrete both. Protein synthesis is accomplished by the ribosomes on the endoplasmic reticulum and transferred first to the cisternae of the endoplasmic reticulum and then to the Golgi apparatus. The Golgi apparatus is the site of carbohydrate synthesis and plays a key role in the elaboration of mucus. In serous cells, the secretory granules discharge their contents by establishing a continuity between membranes of the granule and the apical cell surface. For mucous cells, secretory granules are discharged through gaps in the cell surface.

Innervation

Secretion is controlled by physical and psychic stimulation mediated through the autonomic nervous system. Physical stimuli from the oral cavity and psychic stimuli from taste, smell, or sight centers travel afferent pathways to the superior and inferior salivatory nuclei in the medulla. Both sympathetic and parasympathetic pathways are involved. Parasympathetic innervation of the parotid involves the ninth, seventh, and fifth cranial nerves. Preganglionic fibers leave the inferior salivatory nucleus with the ninth cranial nerve, cross the tympanic cavity with the tympanic plexus (Jacobson's nerve), exit the tympanic cavity as the lesser superficial petrosal nerve, and synapse in the otic ganglion. The postganglionic fibers reach the parotid via the auriculotemporal branch of the third division of the fifth cranial nerve (the nerve implicated in postoperative gustatory sweating, e.g., Frey's syndrome). Parotid sympathetic innervation comes via the ventral roots of the upper three thoracic spinal cord segments, and ascend in the cervical sympathetic chain to the superior cervical ganglion to synapse. Postganglionic fibers travel to the gland with its arterial supply (Figure 1–8).

The submandibular and sublingual glands receive their parasympathetic innervation via the seventh and fifth cranial nerves. Preganglionic fibers leave the superior salivatory nucleus as the nervus intermedius part

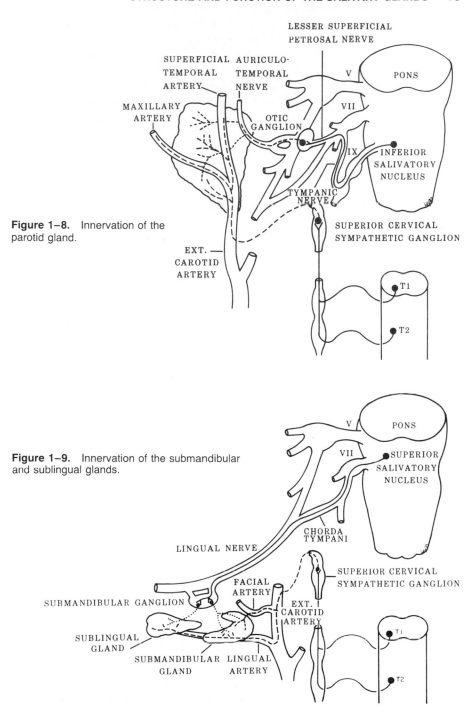

Figure 1–8. Innervation of the parotid gland.

Figure 1–9. Innervation of the submandibular and sublingual glands.

of the seventh cranial nerve, cross the tympanic cavity as the chorda tympani, exit through the petrotympanic fissure, and join the lingual branch of the third branch of the fifth cranial nerve. The fibers synapse in the submandibular ganglion or in small ganglia within the submandibular gland (Langley's ganglion) and travel on to the submandibular or sublingual gland. The ganglion to the submandibular gland must be carefully transected to avoid injury to the lingual nerve in any operative procedure

TABLE 1–2   Factors Affecting Flow Rate and Composition of Saliva

Central Nervous System
   Direct stimulant—cocaine, strychnine, reserpine
   Indirect stimulant—morphine, digitalis, quinidine
   Destructive—encephalitis, mass lesions, cerebrovascular accidents, neurosurgical procedures
   Inhibitors—barbiturates, general anesthetics, antihistamines
Drugs
   Parasympathomimetics, parasympatholytics
   Sympathomimetics, sympatholytics
   Ganglionic blockers
   Miscellaneous—digitalis, muscle relaxants, anti-parkinsonism drugs, theophylline
Loss of Functioning Gland Substance
   Irradiation
   Aplasia
   Chronic inflammation—chronic infection, benign lymphoepithelial lesion, Sjögren's syndrome, sicca syndrome
   Duct obstruction
Hormonal Changes
   Cushing's disease, Addison's disease
   Aldosteronism
   Menstruation, pregnancy
Systemic Diseases
   Alcoholism
   Cystic fibrosis
   Hypertension
   Diabetes mellitus
   Sarcoidosis
   Obesity
   Hyperlipidemia
   Malnutrition
Mucous Membrane Irritation
   Smoking
   Quinine
   Peppermint
Factors Affecting Fluid and Electrolyte Balance
   Diabetes insipidus
   Diuretics
   Dehydration
   Uremia

involving excision of the gland. Sympathetic innervation is similar to that of the parotid, with fibers coming from the carotid plexus to the glands with their respective arterial supplies, the facial and lingual arteries (Figure 1–9). The control of secretion is complex (Table 1–2). Parasympathetic and sympathetic innervation affect acinar cells differently, and the alpha and the beta adrenergic innervation may also have different effects.[5] The autonomic innervation may also affect the duct cells, which are involved in the active transport of electrolytes. Following denervation, reflex salivation ceases and partial atrophy occurs, but the gland becomes more sensitive to epinepherine and acetylcholine. Further, vasoconstriction and vasodilitation may secondarily alter acinar and ductal activity.

BIOCHEMISTRY

Composition of Saliva

Several factors influence the composition of saliva. The collection technique will produce either whole saliva or the secretions of a single gland, and either stimulated or unstimulated saliva. The use of whole saliva obtained by having the subject expectorate into a container is not ideal, because it is impossible to accurately determine the flow rate which alters the concentration of many constituents and because it is contaminated by desquamated cells, food particles, bacteria, and other debris. For practical purposes, submandibular and sublingual saliva can be collected together with little influence on the results, since the sublingual saliva represents only a small percentage. Results vary depending on whether stimulated or unstimulated saliva is collected. For unstimulated saliva, 5 minutes should be allowed after application of the collecting device for the gland to return to its resting state. For stimulated saliva, a standard technique should be used. Sour candy or 2 percent citric acid works well. In either situation, the flow rate should be recorded. The time of day should be standardized (q.v.).

The rate of salivary flow is highly variable. There is a diurnal variation with reduced production in the early morning and increased production in the afternoon.[15] The rate is near zero during sleep, but may reach 4 ml per minute during maximal stimulation. The normal resting parotid flow rate is 0.04 ml per minute per gland; for the submandibular gland the rate is 0.05 ml per minute per gland.[16] Stimulated flow for a single submandibular gland can reach 0.6 ml per minute. The average daily volume has not been well studied and is difficult to measure accurately. The measured daily volume in two patients with esophageal-cutaneous fistulas averaged

500 ml.[17] It is interesting that xerostomia usually is not noted until the average rate drops to less than 0.2 ml per minute per gland.[18] When collecting saliva, it is important to be cognizant of the many local and systemic factors that influence the flow rate or the composition (Table 1–2).

The specific gravity of saliva varies from 1.000 to 1.010, increasing with increasing flow rate. The relative viscosities of the three major salivary glands after stimulation are: parotid, 1.5; submandibular, 3.4; and sublingual, 13.4 centipoises.[19] The viscosity is directly related to the percentage of mucous cells. The pH is slightly acidic prior to secretion into the oral cavity, but becomes slightly alkaline upon entering the oral cavity from loss of CO_2. Since HCO_3 increases with increasing flow rate, the pH becomes elevated at high flow rates. About 90% of the total volume of saliva comes from the parotid and submandibular glands in approximately equal amounts. The minor salivary glands account for about 7 percent,[20] and the sublingual glands contribute the remainder.

The acini secrete an isotonic solution by the active transport of sodium from the intracellular to the intercellular space. This creates an electrochemical gradient across the basement membrane, which results in the formation of an isotonic, sodium-rich, potassium-poor fluid. This is then modified by the striated duct cells. These cells have a morphology similar to the renal proximal tubule cells associated with water transport, and are

TABLE 1–3 Composition of Saliva

Substance	Parotid	Submandibular
mEq/l		
K	20	17
Na	23	21
Cl	23	20
HCO_3	20	18
Ca	2	3.6
Mg	0.2	0.3
HPO_4	6	4.5
mg/dl		
Urea	15	7
Proteins	250	150
Ammonia	0.3	0.2
Uric acid	3	2
Lysozymes	2.3	1.5
Glucose	<1	<1
IgA	4.0	2.0
Amylase	0.1	0.025
Cholesterol	<1	unknown
pH	5.92	5.73

capable of secreting or reabsorbing water, calcium, chloride, bicarbonate, sodium, and potassium. Modification of the fluid occurs principally by the reabsorption of sodium chloride and, to a lesser degree, the secretion of potassium and bicarbonate. Saliva, the final product, consists of a mixture of electrolytes, enzymes, vitamins, immunoglobulins, and other substances.

The mean values of some of the substances found in saliva are shown in Table 1–3. Flow rate can significantly alter some of these values. As flow rate increases, sodium, bicarbonate, and pH increase, while potassium, calcium, phosphate, chloride, urea, and protein decrease. At near maximal flow rates, sodium, calcium, chloride, bicarbonate, protein, and pH increase, while phosphate decreases, and potassium remains unchanged.

Flow rate is altered by the circadian rhythm, by age and diet, as well as by the local and systemic factors listed in Table 1–2. Flow begins shortly after birth, and the resting flow rate increases until age 3 to 5 years, decreases until age 8 to 10, rises slowly until the end of the third decade, and decreases slowly thereafter. Flow rate is stimulated by the ingestion of highly seasoned foods or foods requiring considerable mastication. Some drugs that alter flow rate are listed in Table 1–4.

Other factors influence the composition of saliva independently of the flow rate. A high protein diet raises the urea concentration. The sodium concentration is altered by aldosterone, glucocorticoids, and ACTH. There is a decrease in calcium and sodium and an increase in potassium in submandibular saliva at ovulation as compared to menstruation, which may be an effect of estrogen.[21] There is disagreement on the effect of a high carbohydrate diet on amylase.[22-24] The concentrations of iodide, calcium, and bicarbonate are dependent on the plasma concentration. The concentrations of urea and uric acid are related to the blood levels, and the effectiveness of hemodialysis can be followed by parotid salivary analysis.[25]

Amylase constitutes the main protein in parotid saliva. Amylase activity in the submandibular gland is 20 percent of that in the parotid, and is negligible in the sublingual gland. The major protein constituents of the more mucous-secreting glands are the glycoproteins, especially sialic acid. The submandibular gland produces a heterogeneous group of largely anionic glycoproteins, whereas those of the parotid are largely cationic. Seventy-five per cent of people secrete a glycoprotein named blood group substance in their submandibular and sublingual saliva. Blood group substance is responsible for blood type, and thus blood type can be determined in secretors from salivary analysis. Another glycoprotein produced by the parotid and submandibular glands is secretory piece, which binds two molecules of IgA to stabilize this IgA and form secretory IgA. The IgA

TABLE 1–4 Drugs Affecting Salivary Flow Rate

Mechanism of Action	Drugs
Increased flow	
CNS	Cocaine, strychnine, reserpine morphine, digitalis, quinidine
Mucous membrane irritant	Chloroform, mercury, ether, noxious irritants
Parasympathomimetic	Urecholine, muscarine, mecholyl, neostigmine, physostigmine
Sympathomimetic	Epinephrine, norepinephrine, ephedrine, amphetamines, neosynephrine, B-iso-proterenol, terbutaline, salbutamol
Decreased flow	
CNS	General Anesthetics, barbiturates, antihistamines
Parasympatholytics	Atropine, scopolamine, methartoline, barbiturates, antihistamines, phenothiazines, amytriptyline
Sympatholytic	Phentolamine, αdi-benamine, ergotamine, chlorpromazine propranalol, dichlorisoprenalin
Ganglionic blockers	Hexamethonium, pentolinium, tetraethylammonium, some psychoactive drugs

itself is produced by plasma cells around the intralobular ducts. Secretory IgA has antiviral and antibacterial activity. Other proteins in saliva include lactoferrin, lactic acid dehydrogenase, acid and alkaline phosphatase, and kallikrein (q.v.).

Function of Saliva

The composition of saliva endows it with several important physical and biochemical properties. The mucous layer protects the underlying oral mucosa from local irritants and from dessication. The glycoproteins serve as a lubricant and help the tongue, oral mucosa, and teeth to function smoothly in speaking and swallowing. In addition, the mucus takes a direct, relatively constant course to the oropharynx, sweeping microorganisms and foreign particles with it for destruction and elimination by the gastrointestinal tract.[26]

Saliva protects the teeth. The minerals aid in posteruption maturation. Calcium and phosphate help to prevent enamel dissolution in plaque. The lubricating function reduces wear. The bicarbonate and phosphate exert antibacterial activity within plaque by their buffering ability.

Several substances have more direct antibacterial or antiviral activity. Secretory IgA does not fix complement, but appears able to agglutinate bacteria and make them more readily phagocytized. Some investigators have found elevated levels of IgA in caries-resistant patients; others have not.[27,28] Small amounts of IgG and IgM are also present, and elevated levels have been found in peridontitis and oral candidiasis. However, patients with hypogammablobulinemia do not have an increased incidence of caries or gingivitis.[29]

Lysozymes are found in the saliva from all major glands. They are formed or concentrated in the basal cells of the striated ducts. The lysozymes from different glands have different structures, but all act as a muramidase by hydrolyzing glycopeptides containing muramic acid in bacterial cell walls.[30]

Lactoferrin is an iron-binding protein in saliva that may inhibit bacterial growth by denying them iron.[31] Lactoperoxidase with hydrogen peroxide and thiocyanate ion (the so-called thiocyanate-dependent factors) can inhibit lactobacillus and cariogenic streptococci, and perhaps coliforms.[32] There is disagreement about the presence or absence of a bacteriolytic substance in the saliva of caries-free people.[33–35]

A substance termed nerve growth factor exists in saliva and markedly stimulates nerve tissue growth. It has been reported to be elevated in the serum of children with neuroblastomas.[36]

Changes in Saliva in Disease

Dehydration, hospitalization, mental stress, psychopathic emotional states, fatigue, infection, increased ambient temperature, tranquilizers, ganglionic blockers, and light deprivation cause decreased flow; cigarette smoking, acute stomatitis, heavy metal poisoning, acrodynia, rabies, and ingestion of highly seasoned foods increase flow. Chewing on one side of the mouth increases the flow on that side.[37]

Xerostomia is usually not complained of until flow rate is less than 0.2 ml per minute per gland. Xerostomia may be primary or secondary, and the causes are numerous. In addition to the aforementioned causes, pernicious and iron deficiency anemia, and loss of salivary tissue (from irradiation, infection, Sjögren's syndrome) cause decreased flow. Most causes of xerostomia are systemic in nature; a small but significant percentage remain idiopathic (Table 1–5).

TABLE 1–5   Etiology of Xerostomia in 80 Patients attending Glasgow Dental Hospital

	Etiology	*Number*	*(%)*
Local	Candidiasis	5	
	Miscellaneous	5	(13)
Systemic	Sjögren's syndrome	30	
	Psychogenic plus drugs	12	
	Drug induced	10	(73)
	Anemia	5	
	Endocrine	2	
Idiopathic		11	(13)

From Mason DK, Chisholm DM: Salivary Glands in Health and Disease. Philadelphia, W.B. Saunders Company, 1975.

Numerous systemically administered drugs can be detected in saliva, including iodide, heavy metals, thiocyanate, morphine, clindamycin, and rifampin.[38] The salivary glands are capable of concentrating iodide, but unlike the thyroid, they cannot organify it. Digitalis toxicity causes greatly elevated levels of potassium and calcium, and this study can be used to distinguish between toxicity and therapeutic dosage.[39]

Many disease states affect salivary composition (Table 1–6). In primary aldosteronism, there is a decreased sodium concentration with normal potassium levels. It has been suggested that a sodium/potassium ratio of 0.3 or less is diagnostic, below 0.5 is suggestive, and above 1.0 rules out aldosteronism.[40] The sodium/potassium ratio returns to normal rapidly after removal of the adrenal tumor.[41] The morphologic similarity between salivary striated duct cells and the renal tubular cells has been mentioned, and the sodium-conserving influence of aldosterone would appear to affect both. Low sodium/potassium ratios are also found in Cushing's disease with a mean ratio of 0.5.[42] High ratios occur in Addison's disease with a mean ratio of 5.0. The normal ratio is 1.3. Pregnancy also affects the electrolyte composition. The submandibular calcium concentration is reduced, the sodium concentration is reduced, and the potassium concentration is elevated in both parotid and submandibular saliva in pregnant women as compared with the postpartum levels in the same women.[43]

The salivary glands, like the other exocrine glands, are affected by cystic fibrosis. The submandibular saliva is thickened by increased calcium and calcium precipitable proteins with no change in viscosity.[44,45] Both dialyzable and nondialyzable calcium are increased in submandibular saliva and, to a lesser degree, parotid saliva.[46] Total protein, amylase, lysozyme, and glycoproteins are increased in submandibular but not parotid saliva.[47,48] There is no change in the flow rate in the major glands,[49]

TABLE 1–6 Changes in Saliva in Disease

Variation from Normal	Effect on Saliva
Dehydration, mental stress, psychopathic emotional states, fatigue, infection, increased ambient temperature, tranquilizers, ganglionic blockers, light deprivation	Decreased flow rate
Cigarette smoking, acute stomatitis, heavy metal poisoning, acrodynia, rabies, highly seasoned foods, pernicious anemia, iron deficiency anemia	Increased flow rate
Primary aldosteronism	Decreased sodium with normal potassium
Cushing's disease	Decreased sodium with normal potassium
Addison's disease	Increased sodium with normal potassium
Pregnancy	Decreased sodium, increased potassium
Cystic fibrosis	Increased calcium, protein, amylase, lysozyme, glycoproteins in submandibular saliva
Hyperparathyroidism	Increased calcium and phosphorus
Essential hypertension	Decreased sodium and flow rate
Sarcoidosis	Decreased amylase and kallikrein
	Increased albumin and lysozyme
Acute pancreatitis	Increased amylase
Alcoholic cirrhosis	Increased potassium, amylase, and flow rate
Acute sialadenitis	Increased sodium and potassium
	Decreased phosphate
	Increased glucose, IgG, IgM, IgA, albumin, transferrin, myeloperoxidase, lactoferrin, lysozyme
Irradiation	Increased sodium, chloride, calcium, protein
	Decreased bicarbonate

but there is a significant reduction of flow in the minor glands.[50,51] The high calcium and phosphorus concentrations are associated with increased dental calculus, but not with increased salivary gland calculi.

Thyroid disease and its treatment may affect the saliva. The salivary glands concentrate iodine to 40 times the plasma level.[52,53] The iodine uptake is apparently unrelated to TSH, and there is little difference between euthyroid, hypothyroid, and hyperthyroid states. There is some evidence that hyperthyroidism and radioiodine change saliva in such a way as to promote dental caries, but the mechanism is unknown.[54,55] Hyperparathyroidism leads to increased calcium and phosphorus in saliva, with the levels paralleling the parathormone levels.[56] In essential hypertension, the sodium concentration and the flow rate are decreased.[57] In sarcoidosis, amylase and kallikrein are decreased in saliva,[58] while albumin and lysozyme are increased.[59] After treatment, the albumin and amylase return to normal, but the lysozyme level remains increased. Acute pancreatitis

TABLE 1–7 Changes in Saliva in Sjögren's Syndrome

	Sjögren's	*Controls*
mEq/l		
Sodium	65	23
Chloride	64	23
Potassium	20	22
Phosphate	2.3	6.3
Calcium	1.9	2.1
mg/dl		
Urea	9.8	10.5
ml/min		
Flow rate	0.17	0.58

may cause an increase in amylase. Alcoholic cirrhosis may cause an increased flow rate with increased potassium and amylase.[60] Salivary flow rate is decreased by depression and increased by schizophrenia.[61]

Inflammatory lesions cause several changes in saliva. In acute infections, the sodium and potassium levels approach those of serum.[62] This is probably due to the temporary breakdown of the normal salivary-blood barrier and a toxic effect on the normal transport systems for sodium resorption and potassium secretion.[63] There is also a marked decrease in phosphate, which is peculiar since phosphate is normally inversely related to the flow rate. Other elements that are elevated include glucose, IgA, IgG, IgM, albumin, and transferrin, which leak from plasma, and myeloperoxidase, lactoferrin, and lysozyme, which are produced by the inflammatory infiltrate. IgG dominates the immunoglobulins, reflecting the normal serum pattern rather than the normal salivary pattern, in which IgA dominates. All of the immunoglobulins are in a much higher concentration relative to the albumin in saliva than in blood, suggesting local synthesis by the inflammatory infiltrate. A special inflammatory lesion, Sjögren's

TABLE 1–8 Diseases Causing Diagnostic Compositional Abnormalities

Primary aldosteronism
Cushing's disease
Addison's disease
Pregnancy
Cystic fibrosis
Diabetes mellitus
Osteoporosis
Collagen diseases
Sarcoidosis

TABLE 1–9   Glandosane: Synthetic Saliva (Prof. Dr. J. Matzker)

	gm/l
Carboxymethylcellulose	10.000
Sorbitol	30.000
Potassium chloride	1.200
Sodium chloride	0.843
Magnesium chloride	0.051
Calcium chloride	0.146
Dipotassium hydrogen phosphate	0.342

Composition in mEq/1		mEq/l
Cations:	Na	14.4
	K	21.1
	Mg	0.5
	CA	2.0
Anions:	Cl	33.0
	HPO_4	4.0
	SCN_4	1.0
pH	7.2	
Specific gravity	1.015	
Spray on mucous membranes as needed.		

TABLE 1–10   Artificial Saliva (Erling Johansen, M.D., University of Rochester, New York)

Calcium Solution	
$CaCO_3$	3.275 gm
NaCl	21.576 gm
HCl (5M)	10.000 ml
distilled water	1 gal
Phosphate Solution	
NaF (1000 ppm F)	35.000 ml
$Na_2 HPO_4$	3.119 gm
NaCl	21.576 gm
NaOH (1M)	2.000 ml

The pH is adjusted with additional NaOH or HCl as needed to bring the mixture of equal volumes to pH 6.95. Following tooth brushing, flossing, and application of the acidified fluoride, the patient mixes equal volumes of Ca solution and PO_4 solution and applies it once per day as needed.

TABLE 1–11   Va-Oralube

Reagent	Volume
Rx	
KCl	2.498 gm
NaCl	3.462 gm
$MgCl_2$	0.235 gm
$CaCl_2$	0.665 gm
K_2HPO_4	3.213 gm
KH_2PO_4	1.304 gm
Menthyl p-hydroxybenzoate	8.0 gm
Flavoring	16.0 gm
70% Sorbitol (Sorbo)	171.0 gm
Na carboxy methylcellulose	40.0 gm
NaF	17.68 mg
FD&C Red 40 Dye (2%)	1.0 ml
Water, q.s. ad	4000 ml

syndrome, also causes changes in salivary composition (Table 1–7). Important diseases that cause compositional abnormalities that can be used diagnostically are listed in Table 1–8.

Irradiation causes significant changes in saliva, the most obvious being a marked reduction in flow rate. This leads to a significant increase in dental caries. Numerous authors have shown flow rates to be reduced 95 percent and more after full-course radiation therapy; these rates persist indefinitely.[64,65] Histopathologic studies have shown that the parotid acini and the serous acini from the submandibular gland are severely injured, but there is little discernible change in the mucous cells.[66] As might be expected, the composition is also affected, with increases in sodium, chloride, calcium, and protein and a decrease in bicarbonate.[67]

Artificial Saliva

Artificial saliva is useful in any situation that leads to xerostomia. The most common of these are irradiation, Sjögren's syndrome, and sicca syndrome. Artificial saliva facilitates speech, mastication, and deglutition. It also reduces wear on teeth and promotes mineralization. Three popular formulations are given in Tables 1–9 to 1–11.

REFERENCES

1. Godwin JT: Benign lymphoepithelial lesion of the parotid gland. Cancer 5:1089, 1952.
2. Mesa-Chavez L: Sebaceous glands in normal and neoplastic parotid glands. Possible significance of sebaceous glands in respect to the origin of tumors of the salivary glands. Am J Path 25:627, 1949.

3. Batsakis JG: Tumors of the Head and Neck. Baltimore, Williams & Wilkins, 1979.
4. Emmelin N, Garrett JR, Ohlin P: Neural control of salivary myoepithelial cells. J Physiol 196:381, 1968.
5. Eversole LR: Histogenic classification of salivary tumors. Arch Path 92:433, 1971.
6. Regezi JA, Batsakis JG: Histogenesis of salivary gland neoplasms. Otolaryngol Clin N Am 10:297, 1977.
7. McCormack LJ, Cauldwell EW, Anson BJ: The surgical anatomy of the facial nerve with special reference to the parotid gland. Surg Gynec Obst 80:620, 1945.
8. McCabe BF, Work WP: Parotidectomy with special reference to the facial nerve. In Maloney WH (ed): Otolaryngology. Vol 4. Hagerstown, Harper & Row, 1975, Chap. 9, p. 38.
9. Tabb HG, Tannehill JF: The tympanomastoid fissure: a reliable approach to the facial nerve in parotid surgery. S Med J 66:1273, 1973.
10. Love JT Jr, Marchbanks JR: Injury to the facial nerve associated with the use of a disposable nerve stimulator. Otolaryngology 86:61, 1978.
11. Coleman CC: Results of facio-hypoglossal anastomosis in the treatment of facial paralysis. Ann Surg 11:958, 1940.
12. Crumley RL: Interfascicular nerve repair. Is it applicable in facial injuries? Arch Otolaryngol 106:313, 1980.
13. Conley, J, Baker DC: The surgical treatment of extratemporal facial paralysis: an overview. Head Neck Surg 1:12, 1978.
14. Tucker HM: Restoration of selective facial nerve function by the nerve muscle pedicle technique. Clin Plast Surg 6:293, 1979.
15. Dawes D: Circadian rhythms in human salivary flow rates and composition. J Physiol 220:529, 1972.
16. Shannon IL, Suddick RP, Dowd FT: Salivary Composition and Secretion. Basel, S Karger, 1974.
17. McKeown KD, Dunstone GH: Some observations on salivary secretions and fluid absorption by mouth. Br Med J 2:670, 1959.
18. Mandel ID: Sialochemistry in diseases and clinical situations affecting salivary glands. CRC Crit Rev Clin Lab Sci 12:321, 1980.
19. Schneyer LH: Methods for the collection of separate submaxillary and sublingual saliva in man. J Dent Res 34:257, 1955.
20. Dawes C, Wood CM: The contribution of oral minor mucous gland secretions to the volume of whole saliva in man. Arch Oral Biol 18:337, 1973.
21. Puskulion L: Salivary electrolytes changes during normal menstrual cycle. J Dent Res 51:1212, 1972.
22. Behall KM, Kelsoy JL, Holden JM, Clarke W: Amylase and protein in parotid saliva after load doses of different dietary carbohydrates. Am J Clin Nutr 26:17, 1973.
23. Wesley-Hadziya B, Pigeon H: Effect of diet in West Africa on human salivary amylase activity. Arch Oral Biol 17:1415, 1972.
24. Bates JF: Some observations on the relationship between the concentration of parotid amylase and dietary carbohydrate in human subjects. Br Dent J 112:114, 1962.
25. Shannon IL, Katz KF, Farland M: Parotid fluid urea nitrogen for the monitoring of hemodialysis. N Engl J Med 271:37, 1964.
26. Bloomfield AL: Dissemination of bacteria in the upper air passes. 1. The circulation of foreign particles in the mouth. Am Rev Tuber Pulm Dis 5:903, 1921.
27. Shklaia IF, Revelstad GH, Lamberts BL: A study of some factors influencing phagocytosis of cariogenic streptococci by caries-free and caries-active individuals. J Dent Res 48:842, 1969.
28. Zergo AN, Mandel ID, Goldman R, Khurona HS: Salivary studies in human caries resistance. Arch Oral Biol 16:557, 1971.
29. Brandtzaeg P, Fjellanger I, Djeruldsen ST: Human secretory immunoglobulins. I. Salivary secretions from individuals with normal or low levels of serum immunoglobulins. Scand J Haemotol Suppl 12:3, 1970.
30. Jolles P: Relationship between chemical structure and biological activity of hen egg-white lysozyme and lysozymes of different species. Proc Roy Soc B 167:350, 1967.
31. Masson PL, Heremans JF, Prignot JJ, Wauters G: Immunohistochemical localization and

bacteriostatic properties of an iron-binding protein and bronchial mucus. Thorax 21:538, 1966.

32. Morrison M, Steele WF: Lactoperoxidase, the peroxidase in the salivary gland. In Person P: Biology of the Mouth. Washington D.C., Am Assoc Adv Sci, 1968.

33. Green GE: A bacteriolytic agent in salivary globulin of caries-immune human beings. J Dent Res 38:265, 1959.

34. Green GE: Properties of a salivary bacteriolysin and comparison with serum beta lysin. J Dent Res 45:882, 1966.

35. Geddes DA: Failure to demonstrate the antibacterial factors of Green in caries-free parotid saliva. In MacPhee T: Host Resistance to Commensal Bacteria. Edinburgh, Churchill Livingstone, 1972, pp. 84–89.

36. Burdman JA, Goldstein MN: Long-term tissue culture of neuroblastomas. III. In vitro studies of a nerve growth stimulating factor in sera of children with neuroblastoma. J Nat Cancer Inst 33:123, 1964.

37. Kerr AC: The Physiological Regulation of Salivary Secretions in Man. A Study of the Response of Human Salivary Glands to Reflex Stimulation. Oxford, Pergamon Press, 1961.

38. Wotman S, Mandel ID: Salivary indicators of systemic disease. Postgrad Med 53:73, 1973.

39. Wotman S, Bigger TJ, Mandel ID, Bartlestone HS: Salivary electrolytes in the detection of digitalis toxicity. N Engl J Med 285:871, 1971.

40. Lawler DP, Hickler RB, Thorn GW: The salivary sodium-potassium ratio. N Engl J Med 267:1136, 1962.

41. Wotman S, Goodwin FJ, Mandel ID, Laraugh JH: Changes in salivary electrolytes following treatment of primary aldosteronism. Arch Int Med 124:477, 1969.

42. Frawley TF, Thorn FW: The relation of the sodium-potassium ratio to adrenal cortical activity. In Mote JR (ed): Proceedings of Second Annual ACTH Conference. London, Churchill Livingstone, 1951, pp. 115.

43. Marder MZ, Wotman S, Mandel ID: Salivary electrolyte changes during pregnancy. 1. Normal pregnancy. Am J Obstet Gynec 112:233, 1972.

44. DiSant' Agnese PA, David PB: Research in cystic fibrosis. N Engl J Med 295:481, 1976.

45. Boat RF, Wiesman UN, Pallavicini JC: Purification and properties of the calcium precipitable protein in submaxillary saliva of normal and cystic fibrosis subjects. Pediatr Res 8:531, 1974.

46. Wotman S, Mandel ID, Mercadonte J, Denning CR: Parotid and submaxillary calcium in human cystic fibrosis. Arch Oral Biol 16:663, 1971.

47. Mandel ID, Kutscher AH, Denning CR, Thompson RH Jr, Zegarelli EV: Salivary studies in cystic fibrosis. AM J Dis Child 113:431, 1967.

48. Chernick WS, Eichel HJ, Barbero GH: Submaxillary salivary enzymes as a meausre of glandular activity in cystic fibrosis. J Pediatr 65:694, 1964.

49. Bloomfield J, Rush AR, Allars H, Brown JM: Parotid gland function in children with cystic fibrosis and child control subjects. Pediatr Res 6:574, 1976.

50. Kurscher AH, Denning CR, Zegarelli EV, Eriv A, Phelan J, Ellgood K: Capillary tube tests for minor salivary gland secretion in cystic fibrosis. NY State J Med 68:2812, 1968.

51. Gaerlan PF, Eisenberg RJ, Beck RL, Mandel ID, Denning CR: Quantitation of labial salivary gland function in cystic fibrosis, asthma, and normal subjects. J Dent Res, in press.

52. Masen DK, Harden RMcG, Alexander WD: The salivary and thyroid glands. Br Dent J 122:485, 1963.

53. Harden RMcG, Mason DK: Quantitative studies of iodide excretion in saliva in euthyroid, hypothyroid, and thyrotoxic patients. J Clin Endocrinol 25:957, 1965.

54. Schneyer L, Tanchester D: Some oral aspects of radioactive iodine therapy for thyroid patients. NY J Dent 24:308, 1954.

55. Xhonga FA, Van Herle A: The influence of hyperthyroidism on dental erosions. Oral Surg 36:349, 1973.

56. Weinberger A, Sperling O, DeVries A: Calcium and phosphate in saliva of patient with primary hyperparathyroidism. Clin Chem Acta 50:5, 1974.

57. Niedermeier W, Dreizen S, Stone RE, Spies TD: Sodium and potassium concentrations in the saliva of normotensive and hypertensive subjects. Oral Surg 9:426, 1956.
58. Bhoda KD, McNichol NW, Oliver S, Foran J: Changes in salivary enzymes in patients with sarcoidosis. N Engl J Med 281:877 1969.
59. Beeley JA, Chisolm DM: Sarcoidosis with salivary gland involvement: biochemical studies on parotid saliva. J Lab Clin Med 88:276, 1976.
60. Abelson D, Mandel ID, Kormiol M: Salivary studies in alcoholic cirrhosis. Oral Surg 41:188, 1976.
61. Brown CC: The parotid puzzles: a review of the literature on human salivation and its application to psychophysiology. Psychophysiology 7:66, 1978.
62. Mandel ID, Baurmash H: Sialochemistry in chronic recurrent parotitis: electrolytes and glucose. J Oral Path 9:92, 1980.
63. Burgen ASV: Secretory processes in salivary glands. In Handbook of Physiology. Section 6, Vol 2. Washington D.C., American Physiological Society, 1967, Chap 35.
64. Dreizen S, Daley TE, Drane JB, Brown LR: Oral complications of cancer therapy. Postgrad Med 61:85, 1977.
65. Shannon IL, Starke EN, Wescott WB: Effect of radiotherapy on whole saliva flow. J Dent Res 56:693, 1977.
66. Kashima HK, Kirkham WR, Andrew JR: Post irradiation sialadenitis: a study of the clinical features, histopathologic changes, and serum enzyme variations following irradiation on human salivary glands. Am J Roentgenol 94:271, 1965.
67. Dreizen S, Brown LR, Handler S, Levy BM: Radiation induced xerostomia in cancer patients: effect on salivary and serum electrolytes. Cancer 38:273, 1976.

Chapter Two

THE DIAGNOSTIC WORK-UP

A carefully taken history may uncover important clues to the etiology of the salivary gland disorder. As for any disease, the history should be thorough. Special attention should be paid to other system symptoms that may be related to the salivary gland disorder. Neither the patient nor the referring physician may be aware of the relationship. Salivary gland disorders may be related to a wide variety of other system disorders and each must be carefully evaluated (Table 2–1). Careful questioning about skin, joint, or swallowing abnormalities must be done to check for the possibility

TABLE 2–1 Diseases Associated with Salivary Gland Enlargement

I. Nutritional Deficiency
    Hypovitaminosis A
    Generalized malnutrition
    Pellegra
    Beriberi
II. Hormonal Abnormalities
    Diabetes mellitus
    Hypothyroidism
    Testicular atrophy
    Menopause
    Pregnancy, lactation
III. Metabolic Disorders
    Bacillary dysentery
    Celiac disease
    Ancylostomiasis
    Cardiospasm
    Obesity
    Alcoholic cirrhosis
IV. Others
    Carcinoma of the esophagus
    Sjögren's syndrome
    Sarcoidosis
    Uremia

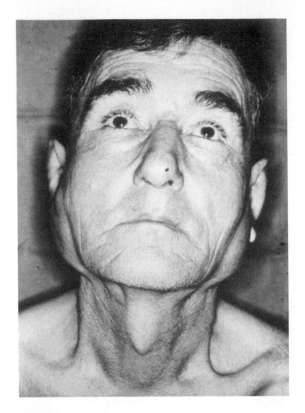

Figure 2–1. Bilateral parotid enlargement in Sjögren's syndrome.

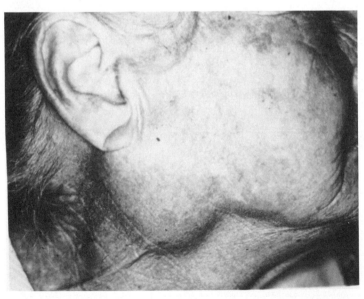

36 Figure 2–2. A pleomorphic adenoma in the tail of the parotid gland.

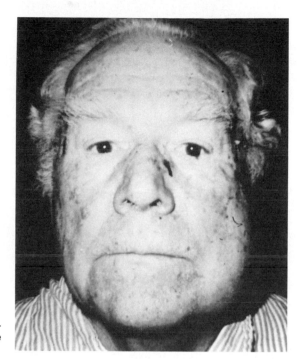

Figure 2–3. Diffuse enlargement of the parotid gland in acute parotitis.

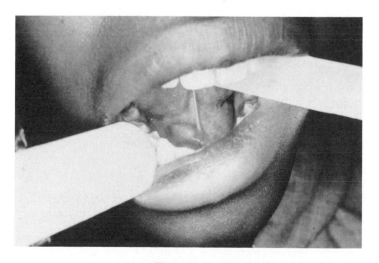

Figure 2–4. Submandibular duct calculus.

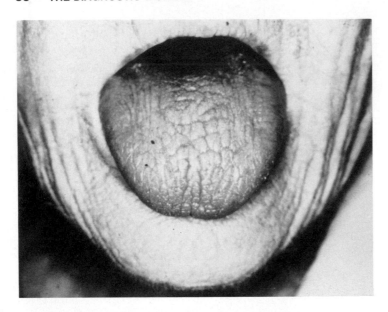

Figure 2–5. Dry tongue in xerostomia in Sjögren's syndrome.

of a collagen disease. A complete endocrinologic evaluation must be done to rule out pituitary, thyroid, gonadal, and pancreatic disorders in particular. Hepatic status must be examined. The lymphoreticular system should be studied. The possibility of metabolic disorders such as diabetes mellitus or hyperlipidemia should be entertained.

A variety of questions must be answered in the evaluation of the salivary glands themselves. First, is more than one gland involved (Figure 2–1)? The vast majority of neoplastic diseases involve a single mass in a single gland (Figure 2–2). There are exceptions, but they are unusual. Is it

TABLE 2–2   Drugs Affecting Salivary Glands

Analgesics	Diuretics
Anticonvulsants	Decongestants
Antiemetics	Expectorants
Antihistamines	Iodine
Antihypertensives	Muscle relaxants
Antinauseants	Central nervous system depressants
Antiparkinsons	Dibenzoxepine derivatives
Antipruritic	Monoamine oxidase inhibitors
Antispasmotics	Phenothiazine derivatives
Appetite suppressants	Tranquilizers
Digitalis	Sedatives

painful? Acute sialadenitis is quite painful (Figure 2–3), whereas many other causes of salivary gland enlargement are not. Does eating affect the disorder? Any obstructive abnormality is apt to cause an increase in discomfort and swelling during alimentation (Figure 2–4). The function of the facial, lingual, and hypoglossal nerves should be questioned. Is there xerostomia (Figure 2–5)? The patient should be questioned regarding allergies, other known illnesses, and medications he is taking. Numerous medications may affect the salivary glands (Table 2–2).

PHYSICAL EXAMINATION

Like the history, the physical examination should be comprehensive. The skin and joints should be examined for evidence of a collagen disease. A careful search should be performed for lymphadenopathy, and the liver, spleen, and thyroid should be palpated. A comprehensive neurologic examination should be conducted.

The local examination depends somewhat on the particular salivary gland involved. The involvement of multiple glands strongly points to a

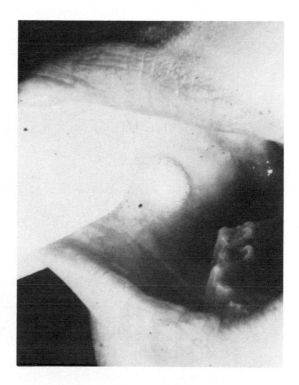

Figure 2–6. Parotid duct calculus.

systemic problem, although there are exceptions. A single mass in a single gland strongly suggests a neoplasm.

Diffuse enlargement of a single gland suggests one of the chronic inflammatory disorders, whereas enlargement of multiple glands suggests Sjögren's syndrome or an endocrinologic or metabolic disorder. The presence of tenderness should be elicited. The major glands should be checked for the character and amount of saliva, and the ducts should be palpated for the presence of a calculus (Figure 2–6). For the parotid gland, all branches of the facial nerve should be checked. For the submandibular and sublingual glands, the hypoglossal and lingual nerves should be evaluated. For a mass in any gland, fixation to bone, skin, or mucosa should be determined.

Care should be taken to avoid confusing a submandibular triangle lymph node with the submandibular gland. A lymph node often is soft-to-firm in consistency, whereas most salivary gland neoplasms, even the benign ones, are hard. In addition, benign lymph nodes usually do not exceed 2 cm in diameter.

In the parotid gland, location of the mass can be a clue to its etiology. Most neoplasms occur in the tail of the gland, beneath the lobule. Lymph nodes rarely occur here and one should always proceed as though the mass were a parotid neoplasm. However, a mass anterior to the tragus may be a lymph node, and may contain metastatic carcinoma. A careful head and neck examination, including the scalp, should be performed. A detailed discussion on metastatic disease to the parotid lymph nodes is presented in the chapter on malignant neoplasms (Chap. 6).

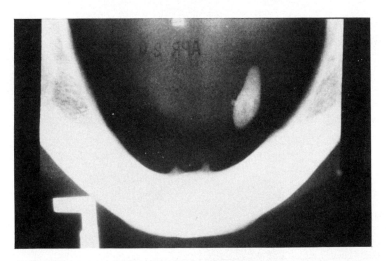

Figure 2–7.   Roentgenogram showing submandibular duct calculus.

If the mass is a parotid neoplasm, palpation may give a clue to the histologic diagnosis. Warthin's tumor is usually soft-to-firm, similar to a lymph node. The pleomorphic adenoma is usually hard, but well circumscribed. One should be quite suspicious of any mass that does not have regular, well-defined borders. These are often malignant.

On occasion sialochemistry can be diagnostically rewarding or confirmatory, and this is discussed in the section on Changes in Saliva in Disease in Chapter 1. Other investigative techniques are generally most useful when only a single gland is involved, particularly a major gland. The following discussion concerns the major techniques used to investigate salivary gland disorders. Plain roentgenography will not be discussed, as its current usefulness is essentially limited to the investigation of radiopaque calculi (Figure 2–7). However, plain roentgenograms are always taken prior to the injection of contrast material during sialography.

SPECIAL RADIOGRAPHIC PROCEDURES

Sialography

Mercury was used for the first sialogram reported in 1904.[1] Both water-soluble and oil-soluble contrast media have been used, with water-soluble media generally being preferred (Table 2–3). Several variations in the technique have been proposed, such as the use of simultaneous xeroradiography[2] and the use of simultaneous pneumography with tomography.[3] The most important variations have been the introduction of secretory sialography[4] and of computed tomographic sialography.[5] The former allows a measure of physiologic evaluation of the gland; the latter is very accurate in identifying mass lesions, both intrinsic and extrinsic (q.v.). Sialography is currently used in the evaluation of calculi, inflammatory lesions, penetrating trauma, and mass lesions involving the major salivary

TABLE 2–3 Comparison of Water-Soluble and Oil-Soluble Contrast Media

	Water-Soluble	Oil-Soluble
Miscible with saliva	4+	0
Physiologic	2+	0
Allergic reaction	0	1+
Opacification	3+	4+
Local reaction	1+	4+
Elimination time	fast	slow

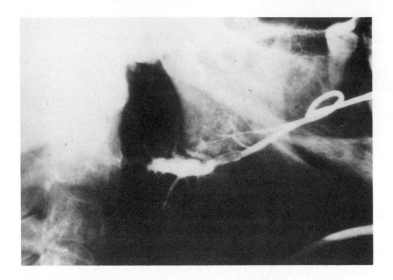

glands. In the normal gland, the parotid duct is approximately 6 cm long and 1 to 3 mm wide with second- and third-order branching. In the lateral view, the duct is approximately 2 cm lateral to the mandible. Accessory glands occasionally are seen superior to the duct. The submandibular duct is 5 cm long and 2 to 4 mm wide with similar branching. Acinar filling may or may not occur, depending on the pressure of injection, the contrast material, and the condition of the gland.

Radiopaque calculi can, of course, usually be seen on the preliminary roentgenograms. Radiolucent calculi are outlined by the contrast medium. Either type may show dilatation of the main duct if it is distal or dilatation of the intraglandular ducts if it is in the hilum[6] (Figure 2–8).

The changes seen in inflammatory lesions depend on the severity and the chronicity of the process. The changes that may be seen include saccular dilatation of the terminal ducts and acini, segmental strictures and dilatation, and pseudocyst formation. It has been reported that some of the changes previously thought to represent sialectasis actually represent extravasation of the contrast material through damaged ducts. Four stages of sialectasis have been described—punctate, globular, cavitary, and destructive. It is the punctate and globular sialectasis that appear to represent extravasation of the contrast material[8] (Figure 2–9).

Sialography can be invaluable in assessing penetrating trauma, especially of the parotid gland. It may demonstrate occlusion of a duct, a

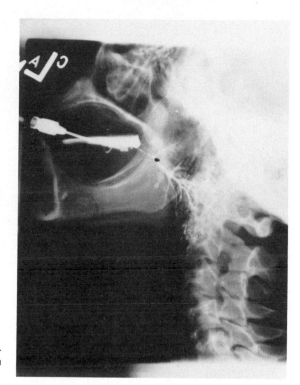

Figure 2–9. Sialogram of parotid showing sialectasis in Sjögren's syndrome.

salivary-cutaneous or salivary-oral fistula, or the development of a sia-locele. Displacement of the gland by edema or a hematoma can also be demonstrated.

Sialography can also supply useful information about some mass lesions. Information can be obtained concerning the size and location of the mass, whether it is intrinsic or extrinsic, and whether it is benign or malignant.[9] Depending on the extent of the lesion and its location, however, this information can be of variable accuracy. Ducts may be draped around or displaced by a mass (Figures 2–10 and 2–11). Infiltrating lesions may disrupt the normal architecture and may cause ductal obstruction or pooling of contrast material. The information that can be obtained is severely restricted if the mass is small or if it is extrinsic to the gland.[10]

Sialography is contraindicated during an acute inflammatory process. Complications are infrequent. Occasional patients experience a foreign body reaction to an oil-soluble contrast solution if there is extravasation. In chronic inflammatory disorders, oil-soluble material may be retained for an extended period.

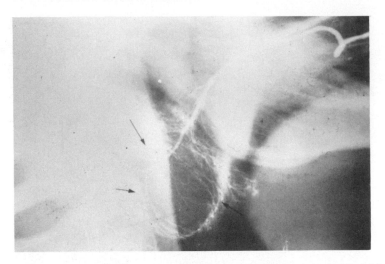

Figure 2–10. Sialogram of parotid showing ducts draped around a Warthin's tumor.

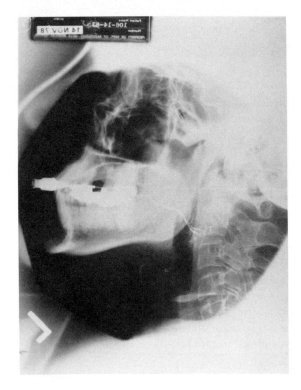

Figure 2–11. Sialogram snowing ducts draped around a pleomorphic adenoma.

Radiosialography

Current radioactive scanning of the major salivary glands is done with technetium. Technetium is an artifically produced radioactive element first manufactured in 1933 by bombarding molybdenum with deuterons. Its atomic number is 43 and its atomic weight is 99. The half-life of its most stable form is 215,000 years, but in the form used medically it is 6 hours. It is used because its tetraoxygenated form, the pertechnetate, is distributed in body fluids as is iodide, except it is not organified in the thyroid. Further, it has no beta radiation and emits gamma radiation at the 140 kev energy level.

Whereas sialography demonstrates the ductal system preferentially, radioisotope scanning is used for evaluation of the parenchyma for mass lesions and for function. Sequential scanning demonstrates the uptake of the pertechnetate from the vascular system and its subsequent secretion in the saliva.[11] Normally the parotid is visible first, followed by the submandibular glands. The glands are generally symmetrical, but not invariably so. Scanning has little to offer in the evaluation of the sublingual and minor salivary glands. The scan should be performed in the resting state as the

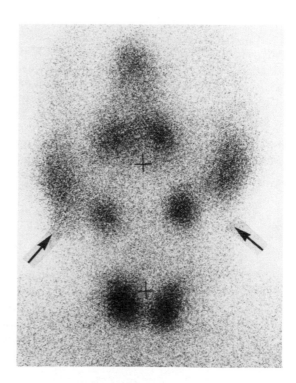

Figure 2–12. Technetium scan of parotids showing Warthin's tumor on the right. Compare the uptake of the arrows.

uptake is greater than in the stimulated state, at least for the parotid.[12] Atropine may be used to block the secretion.

Scintigraphy was first used in the study of mass lesions, especially of the parotid (Figure 2–12). In one excellent study of 106 patients, it was demonstrated that scanning had a 78 per cent accuracy rate. Twenty-two per cent were incorrect and all of these were false-negatives.[13] Smooth-margined radionegative lesions are usually benign tumors or cysts. Irregularly margined radionegative lesions are usually malignant, either primary or metastatic. Smooth-margined radiopositive lesions are usually Warthin's tumor, although the rare oncocytoma also is radiopositive. There has been one report of a pleomorphic adenoma that was radiopositive.[14]

The first report of sequential scintigraphy for physiologic assessment was in 1971.[15] In diseases that affect the salivary parenchyma generally, such as radiation damage or chronic parotitis, the abnormality is evident on sequential scanning by the decreased and delayed uptake.[16]

With the current available techniques, sialography provides more diagnostic information than scanning for either mass lesions or chronic inflammatory disorders.[17] Neither examination is a substitute for a tissue diagnosis in the case of a mass lesion.[18]

Diagnostic Ultrasound

The first report on the use of ultrasound to study salivary glands was in 1971.[19] There are three basic methods of ultrasonic examination of the salivary glands. In the A-mode, the returning sound wave is displayed as a spike on the oscilloscope. In the B-mode, the returning sound wave is displayed as a dot on the oscilloscope. The gray scale, a modfication of the B-mode, allows a greater display of echoes on the oscilloscope to more accurately outline the structure under study. Further, the gain setting can be varied to alter the pattern of the returning sound wave.

In an early study using B-mode with high and low gain settings, it was found that retention cysts and true cysts of the parotid were sonolucent.[20] Benign and malignant tumors appear as solid masses, except for the Warthin's tumor, which is sonolucent at low gain settings, but shows internal echoes at high gain settings. Another study, with histologic follow-up,[21] showed that malignant tumors had a low reflectivity with poorly defined borders. Mixed tumors showed variable reflectivity, but with well-defined borders. Inflammatory lesions showed high reflectivity with diffuse borders. A gray scale study showed improved visualization compared with B-mode; the authors found the technique useful in detecting intrinsic and extrinsic parotid masses.[22] Ultrasound has been used to direct needle aspiration

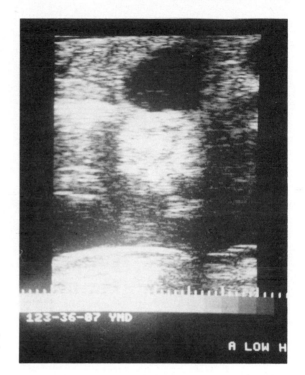

Figure 2–13. Gray scale ultrasound of parotid showing pleomorphic adenoma.

of a parotid abscess,[23] and to locate calculi,[24] but it is yet incapable of reliably separating benign from malignant masses (Figure 2–13).

CT Sialography

Computed tomography with simultaneous sialography was first introduced in 1979.[5] Three additional reports have added to this experience.[25–27] The technique offers no advantage over conventional sialography in the evaluation of inflammatory lesions, but it is unsurpassed in the evaluation of mass lesions. It is able to clearly identify even small lesions that are not palpable, and allows confident differentiation of superficial and deep lobe tumors, as well as intrinsic and extrinsic masses. It is especially useful in differentiating deep lobe tumors and parapharyngeal masses. It clearly shows the proximity of the mass to the facial nerve trunk, and demonstrates extraparotid spread of parotid malignancies. The technique has proven accurate in differentiating benign from malignant neoplasms, with no errors yet reported. The facial nerve should never be

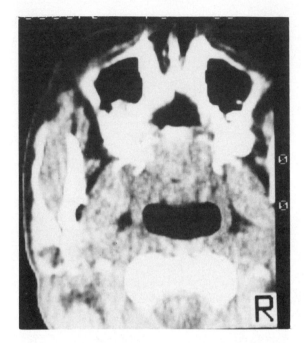

Figure 2–14. CT sialogram showing filling defect in left parotid. This is the pleomorphic adenoma also demonstrated in Figure 2–13.

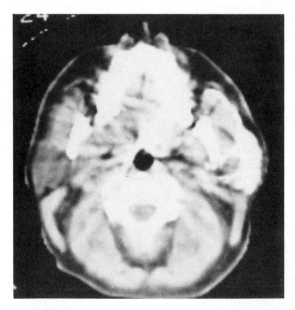

Figure 2–15. CT sialogram demonstrating pleomorphic adenoma in medial aspect of right superficial lobe.

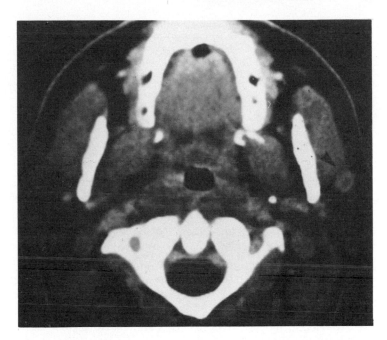

Figure 2–16. CT scan with intravenous contrast enhancement showing mass in right parotid.

sacrificed on the basis of CT sialography, but the study can provide valuable information that may alter the way one prepares the patient preoperatively (Figures 2–14 and 2–15). With the newer generation scanners, many parotid masses can be identified by doing the scan with intravenous contrast enhancement. Sialography is not necessary (Figure 2–16).

FINE NEEDLE ASPIRATION CYTOLOGY

Fine needle aspiration cytology has gained considerable support in recent years as individual institutions have increased their experience. An early report in 1975 showed an 18 per cent change rate from fine needle cytology to the final pathology report.[28] Recent studies show misleading report rates under 10 per cent, with some under 5 per cent. One report of 59 salivary gland lesions had 2 false-positive and no false-negative reports.[29] Another of 51 cases had one false-positive and one false-negative.[30] Another of 62 parotid masses yielded 3 false-positive and no false-negative reports.[31] A very large study of 461 patients gave the following results: exact agreement with the final pathology report in 63 per cent, good and not misleading agreement in 18 per cent, a false report in 8 per cent, and an

TABLE 2–4   Accuracy of Fine Needle Aspiration Cytology

Authors	No. of Patients	False Positive	False Negative
Young et al.[30]	59	2	0
Sismanis et al.[31]	51	1	1
Frable and Frable[32]	62	3	0
Lindberg and Akerman[33]	461	20	20

unsatisfactory specimen in 11 per cent[32] (Table 2–4). In this report, 50 per cent of the false reports involved malignant tumors. Three of 7 acinous cell carcinomas and 4 of 13 mucoepidermoid carcinomas were missed. In one study, electron microscopy to identify the intracellular organelles was added to light microscopy to improve the accuracy rate.[33]

The early criticisms of aspiration cytology centered in three areas. First, since pathologists have difficulty with salivary gland tumors on frozen section, one cannot expect a greater accuracy when there are only a few cells to examine. Clearly, as individual pathologists have gained experience, this criticism has been eliminated for that individual pathologist.

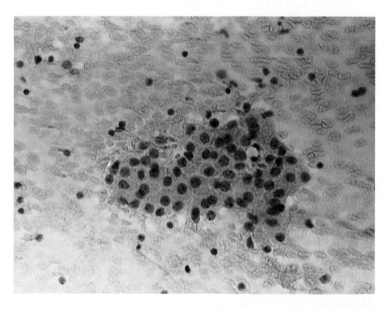

Figure 2–17.   Fine needle cytology showing Warthin's tumor with cluster of oncocytic cells with background of scattered lymphocytes, erythrocytes, and film of granular material. (Courtesy of Britt-Marie Ljung, M.D., Department of Pathology, UCLA School of Medicine.)

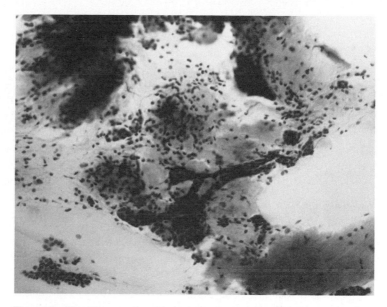

Figure 2–18. Fine needle cytology showing pleomorphic adenoma with clusters of monomorphic epithelial cells and fragments of myxoid stroma with scattered spindle-shaped cells. (Courtesy of Britt-Marie Ljung, M.D., Department of Pathology, UCLA School of Medicine.)

Second, seeding of the tumor may occur along the needle tract. Although this does occur with the Vim Silverman needle, it does not seem to occur with fine-needle aspiration.[34] Third, the tumor may be missed. This certainly can occur, but should be uncommon. In the case of cystic lesions, the return of only acellular fluid does not preclude the presence of a neoplasm.[35] In summary, if the pathologist is experienced in the technique, the accuracy rate should be quite high for pleomorphic adenomas, Warthin's tumors, and metastatic lesions to the parotid[36] (Figures 2–17 and 2–18).

CONCLUSION

As is usual in medicine, a thorough history and physical examination generally brings one to, or near, the diagnosis. It should be clear that the lesion is either inflammatory or a mass. For inflammatory lesions, the single best diagnostic test is the sialogram. Depending on the likely diagnosis, other tests such as a labial biopsy, serologic tests, or culture of the saliva may be indicated.

For space-occupying lesions, the single best test is the CT sialogram, which shows the mass to be either intrinsic or extrinsic and its relationship to the facial nerve. If the mass is cystic or possibly a hemangioma, ultrasound might prove informative. For the solid mass, if the pathologist is experienced, fine-needle aspiration cytology is indicated. Only rarely should therapeutic decisions be made on the basis of fine-needle aspiration cytology. However, the knowledge of the proximity of the mass to the facial nerve, obtained with a CT sialogram, and of the probable histology, obtained with fine-needle cytology, may change the way one prepares the patient preoperatively. Clearly the expected postoperative outcome is different for a benign mixed tumor in the tail of the gland than for an adenoid cystic carcinoma wrapped around the main trunk of the facial nerve.

REFERENCES

1. Carpy A, Poirer P: Traite d'Anatomie Humane. Paris, Masson, 1904, p. 89.
2. Ferguson MM, Davison M, Evans M, Mason WN: Application of xeroradiography in sialography. Int J Oral Surg 5:176, 1976.
3. Granone FG, Juliani G: Submaxillary sialography in combination with pneumoradiography and tomography. Am J Roentgenol 104:692, 1968.
4. Rubin P, Blatt IM: A modification of sialography (preliminary report). Univ Mich Med Ctr Bull 21:57, 1955.
5. Mancuso AA, Rice DH, Hanafee WN: Computed tomography of the parotid gland during contrast sialography. Radiology 132:211, 1979.
6. O'Hara AE: Sialography: past, present, and future. CRC Crit Rev Clin Rad Nucl Med 4:87, 1973.
7. Rubin P, Holt J: Secretory sialography in diseases of the major salivary glands. Am J Roentgenol 77:575, 1957.
8. Som PM, Shugar JM, Train JS, Biller HF: Manifestations of parotid gland enlargement: radiographic, pathologic, and clinical considerations. Part 1. The autoimmune pseudosialectasias. Radiology 141:415, 1981.
9. Gates GA: Current status of radiosialography in tumor diagnosis. Trans Am Acad Ophthalmol Otolaryngol 74:1183, 1970.
10. Calcaterra TC, Hemenway WG, Hansen GC, Hanafee WN: The value of sialography in the diagnosis of parotid tumors. Arch Otolaryngol 103:727, 1977.
11. Greyson ND, Noyak AM: Nuclear medicine in otolaryngological diagnosis. Otolaryngol Clin North Am 11:541, 1978.
12. Stephen KW, Robertson JW, Harden RM: Quantatative aspects of pertechnetate concentration in human parotid and submandibular salivary glands. Br J Radiol 49:1028, 1976.
13. Gates GA: Radiosialographic aspects of salivary gland disorders. Laryngoscope 82:115, 1972.
14. Hendra R, Stebner FC: Evaluation of parotid gland masses by rectilinear scanning. J Oral Surg 33:838, 1975.
15. Schall GE, Anderson LG, Buchignani JS, Wolf RO: Investigation of major salivary duct obstruction by sequential salivary scintigraphy, report of three cases. Am J Roentgenol Rad Ther Nucl Med 113:655, 1971.
16. Eneroth CM, Ling MG: Radiosialometry. II. The diagnostic accuracy of different evaluation parameters. Acta Otolaryngol 81:141, 1976.
17. Schmitt G, Lehmann G, Strotges MW, Wehmer W, Reinecke V, Teske HJ, Rottinger EM: The diagnostic value of sialography and scintigraphy in salivary gland disease. Br J Radiol 49:326, 1976.

18. Gates GA: Sialography and scanning of the salivary glands. Otolaryngol Clin North Am 10:379, 1977.
19. Bogin YN, Romacheva IS, Nakhutina EM: Biolocation diagnosis of diseases of parotid and submaxillary salivary glands. Stomatologia 50:27, 1971.
20. Neiman HL, Phillips JF, Jaques DA, Brown TL: Ultrasound of the parotid gland. J Clin Ultrasound 4:11, 1976.
21. Baker S, Ossoinig KD: Ultrasonic evaluation of salivary glands. Trans Am Acad Ophthalmol Otolaryngol 84:750, 1977.
22. Gooding GA: Gray scale ultrasound of the parotid gland. AJR 134:469, 1980.
23. Magaram D, Gooding GA: Ultrasonic guided aspiration of parotid abscess. Arch Otolaryngol 107:549, 1981.
24. Pickrell KL, Trought WS, Shearin JC: The use of ultrasound to localize calculi within the parotid gland. Ann Plast Surg 1:542, 1978.
25. Som PM, Biller HG: The combined CT-sialogram. Radiology 135:387, 1980.
26. Rice DH, Mancuso AA, Hanafee WN: Computerized tomography with simultaneous sialography in evaluating parotid tumors. Arch Otolaryngol 106:472, 1980.
27. Stone DN, Mancuso AA, Rice DH, Hanafee WN: Parotid CT sialography. Radiology 138:393, 1981.
28. Conley JJ: Salivary Glands and the Facial Nerve. New York, Grune and Stratton, 1975.
29. Young JE, Archibald SD, Shier KJ: Needle aspiration cytologic biopsy in head and neck masses. Am J Surg 142:484, 1981.
30. Sismanis A, Merriam JM, Kline TS, Davis RK, Shapshay SM, Strong MS: Diagnosis of salivary gland tumors by fine needle aspiration biopsy. Head Neck Surg 3:482, 1981.
31. Frable WJ, Frable MA: Thin needle aspiration biopsy: the diagnosis of head and neck tumors revisited. Cancer 43:1541, 1979.
32. Lindberg LG, Akerman M: Aspiration cytology of salivary gland tumors: diagnostic experience from six years' of routine laboratory work. Laryngoscope 86:584, 1976.
33. Hagelgvist E: Light and electron microscopic studies on material obtained by fine needle biopsy. Acta Otolaryngol (Supl) 354:1, 1978.
34. Yamaguchi KT, Strong MS, Shapshay SM, Soto E: Seeding of parotid carcinoma along Vim-Silverman needle tract. J Otolaryngol 8:49, 1979.
35. Zayicek J, Eneroth CM, Jakobson P: Aspiration biopsy of salivary gland tumors. VI. Morphologic studies on smears and histologic sections from mucoepidermoid carcinoma. Acta Cytol 20:35, 1976.
36. Kline TS, Merriam JM, Shapshay SM: Aspiration biopsy cytology of the salivary gland. AM J Clin Pathol 76:263, 1976.

Chapter Three

INFLAMMATORY DISORDERS

ACUTE SUPPURATIVE SIALADENITIS

Acute suppurative sialadenitis may involve the parotid or subman-dibular gland and was first reported in 1828, but the vast majority of cases occur in the parotid gland. The parotid is believed to be more susceptible because parotid saliva has less bacteriostatic activity than submandibular saliva,[1] presumably because the bacterial aggregating ability, and thus eliminating ability, is greater with the high-molecular-weight glycopro-teins in the mucous acini, since the other antibacterial systems seem the same.[2]

Acute suppurative sialadenitis accounts for approximately 0.03 per cent[1,3] of hospital admissions. Thirty to 40 per cent occur in the postopera-tive patient, usually 3 to 5 days postoperative, with the highest incidence following gastrointestinal procedures. The primary pathogenic event is thought to be salivary stasis, either from obstruction or from decreased production of saliva. An ascending bacterial infection occurs and leads to suppuration within the gland. This theory of retrograde infection was first promoted by Cruveilheir in 1836.[4] Predisposing conditions include calculi, duct stricture, dehydration, and poor oral hygiene. These conditions usu-ally exist in a patient with reduced resistance, in a hospital environment, and receiving multiple medications with probably altered oral flora.[5] Many medications further reduce salivary flow.[6] If, in addition, the patient is not eating, he loses the stimulatory effect of mastication on the salivary glands plus the detergent action of food itself. This complication occurs in one in 1000 to 2000 operative procedures. It occurs most frequently in the sixth and seventh decades, although all ages have been reported.[7] The sex distribution is equal.

The classic clinical presentation is the debilitated or postoperative patient who develops acute suppurative parotitis. There is diffuse enlarge-ment of the involved gland with associated induration and tenderness. Purulent saliva can be expressed from the duct orifice. It is bilateral in 20 per cent of cases.[8] The purulent saliva should be cultered for aerobic and anaerobic bacteria and a Gram stain obtained. The offending organism is usually coagulase-positive *Staphlococcus aureus*. Other occasionally im-

55

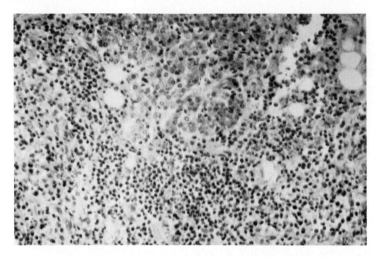

Figure 3–1. Photomicrograph showing acute suppurative parotitis.

plicated aerobic organisms include *Streptococcus pneumonia, Escherichia coli,* and *Haemophilus influenzae.*[9] Anaerobic organisms include *Bacteroides melaninogenicus* and *Streptococcus micros.*[10] The microscopic picture is that of glandular destruction with abscess formation. There is erosion of the ducts with penetration of the exudate into the parachyma (Figure 3–1).

Initial treatment consists of adequate hydration, good oral hygiene, repeated message of the gland, and intravenous administration of the appropriate antibiotic. While awaiting culture results, empiric administration of a penicillinase-resistant, antistaphylococcal antibiotic is advisable, if the Gram stain shows gram-positive cocci. The antibiotic can be changed as indicated by culture results as they are obtained. Quoted mortality rates approach 20 per cent,[11] although much of this is probably because it occurs in the already seriously ill patient. Thus, if a response to the appropriate treatment regimin does not occur quickly, incision and drainage should be performed. This is done by raising a parotid flap as for a parotidectomy, and then using a hemostat to make multiple openings into the gland, spreading in the general direction of the facial nerve. Following this, a drain is placed over the gland and the wound closed. Successful needle aspiration guided by ultrasound has been reported (see section on Ultrasound in Chapter 2).

CHRONIC, RECURRENT SIALADENITIS

Like acute suppurative sialadenitis, the primary pathogenic event in chronic sialadenitis is believed to be a decreased secretion rate with subsequent stasis. Two theories of initiation are currently espoused. One is that repeated acute episodes or a single severe episode of suppurative sialadenitis leads to ductal metaplasia of mucus-secreting glands. This leads to an increased mucus content in the saliva, which contributes to the salivary stasis. The other is that if the gland is colonized by pyogenic bacteria, an acute suppurative infection will result, whereas colonization with opportunistic oral flora will lead to chronic, recurrent sialadenitis. Some cases seem to progress from the recurrent parotitis of childhood.[12] Some of these patients subsequently develop Sjögren's syndrome.[13,14] This disease is much more common in the parotid gland, presumably because of its longer, narrower duct,[15] making it more susceptible to stasis. As time passes, the disease leads to sialectasia, ductal ectasia, and progressive acinar destruction combined with a lymphocytic infiltrate. Histologically it is difficult to differentiate the various types of chronic salivary inflammation. Salivary tissue appears to have a limited tissue response.[16] In general, the sialographic appearance parallels the degree of histologic change, and all chronic inflammatory lesions give similar sialographic and histologic pictures. As important as ductal metaplasia and increased mucus production is acinar destruction. "The mechanism which resists retrograde infection of salivary parenchyma by mouth organisms can operate successfully in the face of increased pressure gradients . . . as long as the normal complement of acinar tissue is available and sufficiently productive to wash the organisms out of the duct."[17] This seems self-evident. The lymphocytic infiltrate is a response to ductal and acinar damage, with progressive replacement of secreting glandular elements by the infiltrate (Figure 3–2).

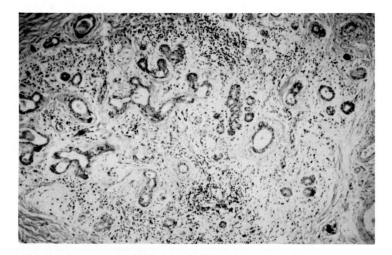

Figure 3–2. Photomicrograph showing chronic parotitis with destruction of the acini, an inflammatory infiltrate, and ductal ectasia.

This progressive glandular destruction causes changes in the chemistry of saliva. Rausch was the first to note increased salivary sodium (> 20 mEq/1) and protein (> 400 mg per cent) in chronic sialadenitis; these values remain normal in noninflammatory enlargement.[18] During acute exacerbations, the sodium and chloride values approach those of serum.[19] A breakdown of the normal salivary-blood barriers and a possible toxic effect on the normal transport systems for sodium resorption and potassium secretion are probably responsible.[20] There is also a marked decrease in the phosphate concentration, particularly since phosphate is normally inversely related to flow rate. Glucose is also considerably elevated, but rapidly returns to normal. Also increased are IgA, IgG, IgM, albumin, and transferrin, which leak from plasma, and myeloperoxidase, lactoferrin, and lysozyme, which are produced by the inflammatory infiltrate or the acini. The IgG dominates the immunoglobulins, reflecting the serum pattern rather than the usual salivary pattern with IgA dominance. The single most prominent salivary protein in acute exacerbations is lactoferrin.[21] The high levels of sodium, albumin, and lactoferrin combined with the low level of potassium will differentiate an acute exacerbation of parotitis from sialosis. Even during quiescent periods, the sodium, albumin, and lactoferrin remain elevated, while there is a normal potassium and a decreased phosphate.

Clinically the patient gives a history of recurrent, mildly painful parotid enlargement, usually associated with eating. Physical examination confirms this, and massage of the gland often produces scanty saliva at the duct orifice. Eighty per cent of patients develop permanent xerostomia. Treatable predisposing factors, such as a calculus or a stricture, should be investigated and, if found, treated appropriately. If none is found, treatment should be otherwise conservative. This would include the use of sialogogues, massage, and antibiotics during acute suppurative exacerbations. If conservative measures fail, and this is unusual, other treatment options include periodic ductal dilatation, ligation of the duct, total gland irradiation, tympanic neurectomy, and excision of the gland. All of these options, except the last, work occasionally, but not uniformly. Ligation of the duct may successfully cause atrophy of the gland, but occasionally results in an acute infection or in a mucocele. Irradiation produces an initial acute inflammatory reaction, but continued treatment results in destruction of the gland. This should only be considered in the older patient, in whom the risk of irradiation-induced carcinoma is reduced. If all else fails, excision of the gland is curative.[22] This can be a difficult operation with considerable oozing of blood, making identification of the facial nerve difficult. Much of this can be reduced by the injection of dilute epinephrine into the incision line and into the area of the main trunk of the facial nerve. Hypotensive anesthesia may prove helpful.

Recurrent parotitis may also involve children from infancy to age 12 and is a somewhat different entity. Unlike the adult form, this form affects more males than females. The underlying cause is unproved, but the disease begins with the sudden onset of either unilateral or bilateral parotid swelling. Attacks may be single or recurrent, with varying degrees of enlargement during and between acute episodes. Saliva may be clear or flocculent, with decreased flow. Salivary chemistries are altered as in the adult form.

Clinically the child usually is not ill, although there may be a mild elevation in the temperature and the white blood cell count. Mild pain may be present, but the child does not complain of xerostomia.[23] The disease may disappear at puberty or continue into adulthood.

BENIGN LYMPHOEPITHELIAL LESION

The benign lymphoepithelial lesion belongs in the spectrum of diseases involving a lymphoreticular infiltration into the gland, combined with acinar atrophy and ductal metaplasia ending in the epimyoepithelial island.[24] The histologic picture is that of chronic inflammation with variations being related only to distribution and severity (Figure 3–3). Some regard this lesion as "end-stage" chronic recurrent parotitis.[25] Other diseases within this spectrum include primary and secondary Sjögren's syndrome. Unlike these, however, the benign lymphoepithelial lesion usually affects only a single salivary gland and has a smaller female predominance.

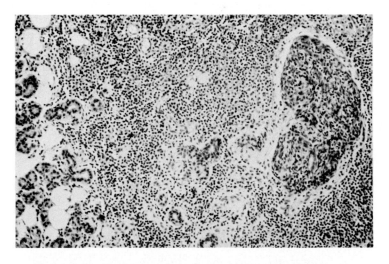

Figure 3–3. Photomicrograph of a benign lymphoepithelial lesion.

TABLE 3–1 Relationship of the Benign Lymphoepithelial Lesion to Other Disorders

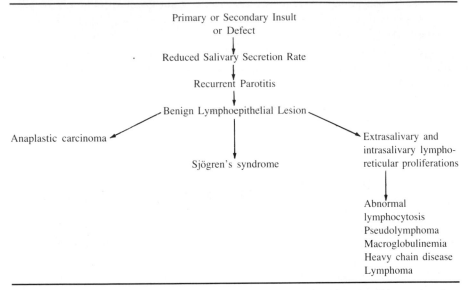

Adapted from Batsakis JG, Sylvest V: Pathology of the Salivary Glands. Chicago, American Society of Clinical Pathologists, 1977.

Evidence that this is a less highly developed form of Sjögren's syndrome is limited and debatable.[26]

It usually begins as an asymptomatic enlargement unless there is superimposed infection. If the lesion is asymptomatic and not cosmetically objectionable, no treatment is necessary. If the lesion is cosmetically unacceptable, the gland may be excised. If intermittent infections occur, they should be treated as acute sialadenitis. Usually massage, sialogogues, and a penicillinase-resistant antibiotic suffice.

Of more concern is the occasional benign lymphoepithelial lesion that evolves into a more aggressive lesion. As of 1980, there had been reported evolution of the disease into 84 cases of lymphoproliferative disease, 27 cases of carcinoma, and 12 cases of pseudolymphoma. The lymphoproliferative disorders are virtually all histiocytic or lymphocytic lymphoma involving extrasalivary sites. The sudden development of hypogammaglobulinemia or leukopenia may herald the onset of lymphoma. The carcinomas are usually salivary and usually anaplastic. Many have been of Indian or Eskimo extraction, but this may represent merely a reporting artifact.[29] These entities should be watched for and treated early and aggressively if they occur. Table 3–1 shows the relationship of the benign lymphoepithelial lesion to the other disorders mentioned.

SJÖGREN'S SYNDROME

Sjögren's syndrome is characterized by a lymphocyte-mediated destruction of the exocrine glands leading to xerostomia and keratoconjunctivitis sicca. It is the second most common autoimmune disease after rheumatoid arthritis.[30] Ninety per cent occur in women. It occurs, but is less common, in children.[29] The average age of occurrence is 50 years.

The clinical manifestations were first described by Hadden in 1888.[31] Four years later, Mikulicz published a single case report of a patient with bilateral lacrimal, parotid, and submandibular gland swelling.[32] In 1933, Sjögren, a Swedish ophthalmologist, published the classic monograph on the disease and emphasized the systemic nature of the disease.[33] In 1953, Morgan and Castleman demonstrated that the histologic findings in Sjögren's syndrome and Mikulicz's disease were identical.[34] Sjogren's syndrome occurs in two forms—primary, which involves exocrine glands only, and secondary, which is associated with a definable autoimmune disease, usually rheumatoid arthritis.[35]

Sjögren's syndrome generally runs a relatively benign course manifesting primarily exocrine gland dysfunction. This leads to burning oral discomfort and a "sandy" sensation in the eye. Either unilateral or bilateral salivary gland swelling, usually involving the parotid, occurs in 80 per cent of primary and 30 to 40 per cent of secondary cases. The swelling may be intermittent or permanent. Arthritis is the most frequent first complaint in secondary Sjögren's.[35] Recent studies have shown that there are genetic differences between primary and secondary Sjögren's syndrome.[36,37] Associated symptoms are numerous and include interstitial pneumonitis, dryness of the skin, Raynaud's phenomenon, achlorhydria, hepatosplenomegaly, genital dryness, hyposthenuria, myositis, and pancreatitis. Patients with primary Sjögren's have a greater incidence of recurrent parotitis, Raynaud's phenomenon, purpura, lymphadenopathy, myositis, and renal involvement than do those with secondary Sjögren's.[38]

TABLE 3–2 Autoimmune Antibodies in Sjögren's Syndrome

Antibody	% Present
Rheumatoid factor	70–90
Antinuclear antibody	55–70
Salivary duct antibody	65
Parietal cell antibody	27
Thyroglobulin antibody	18
Thyroid microsomal antibody	21

A number of laboratory findings suggest that one of the underlying defects in Sjögren's syndrome is B-cell hyper-reactivity, with or without abnormalities of immunoregulation. These include polyclonal hypergammaglobulobulinemia, numerous autoimmune antibodies, both organ- and nonorgan-specific, as well as circulating IgG immune complexes.[39,40] Rheumatoid factor is detectable in 70 to 90 per cent, antinuclear antibody in 55 to 70 per cent, salivary duct antibody in 65 per cent, parietal cell antibody in 27 per cent, thyroglobulin antibody in 18 per cent, and thyroid microsomal antibody in 21 per cent. Elevated levels of antibody to secretory IgA have been reported.[41]

In addition to the B-cell hyper-reactivity, patients with extraglandular Sjögren's syndrome have a markedly decreased proportion of T-cells with an Fc receptor for IgG (T_G),[42] which is reversible with the removal of blocking antibodies.

The sialographic abnormalities parallel the clinical and histologic severity of the disease, with the characteristic lesion being one of varying degrees of sialectasis. Four stages of sialectasis have been described— punctate, globular, cavitary, and destructive.[43] It has recently been demonstrated that the radiographic appearances of punctate and globular sialectasis really represent extravasation of the contrast material through the ducts and not true sialectasis[44] (Figure 3–4).

Grossly and histologically the individual salivary gland resembles the gland involved with chronic inflammation. There is ductal ectasia (or pseudo-ectasia—q.v.) on sialography and lymphoreticular infiltration,

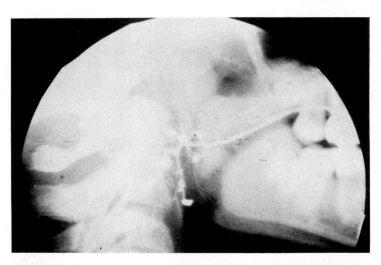

Figure 3–4. Parotid sialogram showing the typical changes of Sjögren's syndrome.

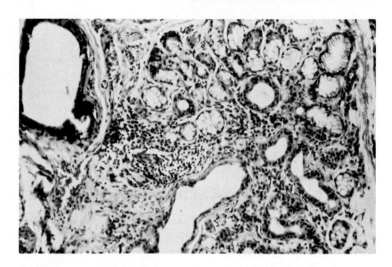

Figure 3–5. Photomicrograph of a labial salivary gland biopsy showing the inflammatory infiltrate and ductal ectasia typical of Sjögren's syndrome.

acinar destruction, and the formation of epimyoepithelial islands on histology. The lymphoreticular infiltrate appears to consist largely of small or medium-sized lymphocytes and plasma cells on electron microscopy.[45] Sjögren's syndrome involves the minor salivary glands in 70 per cent of patients,[46] and the diagnosis can be made by labial, nasal mucosa, or palate biopsy. This is the simplest way of confirming the clinical diagnosis (Figure 3–5).

Sialochemical studies have revealed a number of abnormalities (Table 3–3). It has been reported that parotid lysozyme is elevated,[47] while lacri-

TABLE 3–3 Sialochemical Values in Sjögren's Syndrome

Parameter	Sjögren's	Controls
Flow rate (ml/min)	0.17	0.58
Sodium mEq/l	65	23
Chloride mEq/l	64	23
Potassium mEq/l	20	22
Phosphate mEq/l	2.3	6.3
Calcium mEq/l	1.9	2.1
Urea mEq/l	9.8	10.5
Total protein	252	236
IgA	5.8	3.6
IgG	1.0	0.5
Albumin	1.3	0.8
Amylase (units/ml)	1480	1440

mal lysozyme is decreased.[48] Sodium and chloride concentrations are approximately three times normal, while the phosphate level is one-half normal.[49] Experimental evidence appears to show that the metaplastic ductal cells are incapable of the active resorption of sodium and chloride.[50] The potassium is usually normal, as in chronic inflammatory disorders. The amylase and total protein concentrations are normal, suggesting that the remaining acinar cells are capable of normal protein synthesis. The greatly decreased flow rate, however, markedly reduces the amount of antibacterial material delivered to the oral cavity. Dental caries are significantly increased.[51]

Sjögren's syndrome, like the benign lymphoepithelial lesion, is associated with an increased incidence of lymphoma. The incidence is increased 44 times over the normal and is usually of the histiocytic or mixed histiocytic-lymphocytic type.[52] Fifty per cent of those who develop a lymphoma have had prior irradiation to the parotid. Pseudolymphoma may also occur and, like the lymphoma, has been shown to be of B-cell origin.[53,54] Sjögren's syndrome has also been associated with biliary cirrhosis,[55] other liver abnormalities,[56] involvement of the larynx,[57,58] the development of membranous glomerulonephritis,[59] autoimmune liver disease,[60] and secondary amyloidosis.[61]

Treatment is symptomatic. The xerostomia leads to a burning oral discomfort, difficulty in eating dry foods, and decreased taste sensitivity. There may be mucosal ulceration and increased dental caries. The simplest treatment is the use of an artificial saliva swirled in the mouth and swallowed every 3 to 4 hours (see Chap. 1). In addition the salivary glands can be stimulated to produce what saliva they can. Eating 3 to 4 raw apples per day is excellent for this, as is sour candy. Dental hygiene must be impeccable. Acute infections should be treated as acute sialadenitis.

Xerophthalmia is best treated with artificial tears such as ¼ per cent hydroxycellulose drops every 3 to 4 hours as needed. Taping the lids closed at bedtime is an excellent precaution. Occasionally tarsorrhaphy may be necessary. Care must be taken to prevent corneal ulcerations and perforations, which have been reported.[62] These patients also have an increased incidence of otitis media, bronchitis, pneumonia, pancreatitis, and atrophic gastritis, which should be watched for and treated appropriately.

It has been suggested that an inadequate synthesis of prostaglandin E1 is the key factor in the xerostomia and xerophthalmia, and some success in raising tear and saliva production has been reported by raising the level of prostaglandin E1 precursors and vitamin C in the diet.[63] Some have recommended the use of immunosuppressive agents in the hopes of avoiding the development of a subsequent malignancy.[64] With this regimen, lymphocytic infiltration has been reversed.[65]

GRANULOMATOUS DISEASES

Primary tuberculosis of salivary tissue is uncommon. It usually involves the parotid gland, is usually unilateral, and is believed to arise from a focus in the tonsils or teeth. It may occur in one of two forms—an acute inflammatory lesion or a chronic tumorous lesion. The former is a difficult diagnostic problem. The diagnosis often is not made until, faced with a lack of response to conventional antibiotics, an acid-fast salivary stain and a PPD are performed. The PPD may be unreliable, as infections caused by the atypical mycobacteria are increasing relative to *Mycobacterium tuberculosis hominis.*[66,67] Treatment is as for any acute tuberculosis infection. The latter disease is usually diagnosed only after excision of the gland for a suspected tumor. The excision is curative. Secondary infections can occur, but involve the submandibular or sublingual glands more frequently than the parotid.

Animal scratch disease may involve the salivary glands, but only by contiguous spread from a lymph node. This is a self-limiting disease and treatment is symptomatic.

Actinomycosis may also occur in the salivary glands. Treatment involves incision and drainage combined with long-term penicillin therapy as with actinomycosis elsewhere.

Sarcoidosis is a granulomatous disease of cryptogenic etiology that is a diagnosis of exclusion (Figure 3–6). While salivary gland involvement

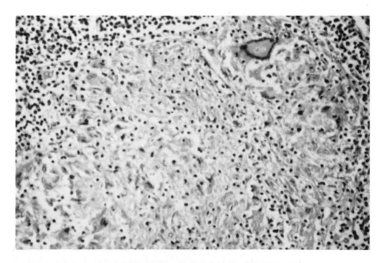

Figure 3–6. Photomicrograph of sarcoidosis showing the noncaseating granuloma and the inflammatory infiltrate.

occurs in 33 per cent of cases in histologic studies,[68] it is clinically manifest in only 6 per cent.

Uveoparotid fever (Heerfordt's syndrome) is a particular form of sarcoidosis that manifests uveitis, parotid swelling, and facial paralysis. It usually occurs in the third or fourth decade and begins with a prodrome of fever, malaise, weakness, nausea, and night sweats lasting several days to several weeks. This may occur with or without other systemic manifestations of sarcoidosis. Generally both parotids enlarge simultaneously, and submandibular, sublingual, and lacrimal involvement may occur. The swelling lasts months to years without suppuration and with eventual resolution. Involvement of the minor salivary glands may occur, and labial biopsy may establish the diagnosis.[69]

The sialographic appearance depends on the extent of glandular invasion and ranges from normal to moderate loss of ductal radicals. Technetium scanning is frequently abnormal.[70] Histologic examination reveals the expected noncaseating granulomas, which, like tuberculosis, involve the lymphoid tissue more than the parenchyma.[71] Sialochemistry reveals a decrease in amylase and kallikrein,[72,73] with an increase in albumin and lysozyme.[74]

Treatment is symptomatic, with corticosteroids being most useful in the acute phase, particularly for the facial paralysis. Even without treatment, the facial paralysis is usually transient. The uveitis should be followed closely as it can lead to glaucoma.

VIRAL INFECTIONS

Mumps is by far the most common cause of parotid swelling and is the most common viral agent to involve the salivary glands. It is most commonly recognized in the 4- to 6-year-old age group. The incubation period is 2 to 3 weeks, with a clinical onset characterized by pain and swelling in one or both parotids. Systemic symptoms include fever, malaise, myalgias, and headache, and usually resolve before the parotid swelling. Many cases, however, are subclinical, and studies have shown that greater than 95 per cent of adults have neutralizing antibodies.[75] The diagnosis is made by demonstrating antibodies to the mumps S and V antigens and to the hemagglutination antigen.[76] The virus may also be isolated from the urine from 6 days before until 13 days after the salivary gland symptoms. Major complications include sudden deafness, pancreatitis, meningitis, and orchitis. Islet cell antibodies have been reported,[77] and a recent epidemiologic study has shown a statistically significant association between mumps and the subsequent rapid onset of childhood diabetes.[78]

Salivary gland inclusion disease is a rare form of cytomegalic inclu-

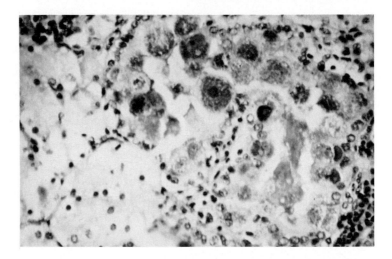

Figure 3–7. Photomicrograph of cytomegalic inclusion disease.

sion disease (Figure 3–7). It involves newborns and may cause mental and physical retardation as well as hepatosplenomegaly, jaundice, and thrombocytopenic purpura. Other viral agents that may infect the salivary glands include Coxsackie A, ECHO, influenza A, and the virus of lymphocytic choriomeningitis. The treatment in all cases is symptomatic.

REFERENCES

1. Spratt J: Etiology and therapy of acute pyogenic parotitis. Surg Gynec Obst 112:391, 1961.
2. Mandel ID: Sialochemistry in diseases and clinical situations affecting salivary glands. CRC Crit Rev Clin Lab Sci 12:321, 1980.
3. Bronson B, Kugel C, Stafford C, Morel E: The re-emergence of postoperative parotitis. West J Surg Obst Gynec 67:38, 1959.
4. Cited in Berdnt R, Buck R, Buxton R: The pathogenesis of acute suppurative parotitis. Am J Med Sci 182:639, 1931.
5. Lundgren A, Kylen P, Odkvist LM: Nosocomial parotitis. Acta Otolaryngol 82:275, 1976.
6. Krippaehne W, Hunt T, Dunphy J: Acute suppurative parotitis. Ann Surg 156:251, 1962.
7. Banks WW, Handler SD, Glade GB, Turner HD: Neonatal submandibular sialadenitis. Am J Otolaryngol 1:261, 1980.
8. Schwartz A, Devine K, Beahrs O: Acute postoperative parotitis. Plast Reconstr Surg 25:51, 1960.
9. Fainstein V, Musher DM, Young EJ: Actue bilateral suppurative parotitis due to Haemophilus influenzae. Report of two cases. Arch Intern Med 139:712, 1979.
10. Anthes WH, Blaser MJ, Reller LB: Acute suppurative parotitis associated with anaerobic bacteremia. Am J Clin Pathol 75:160, 1981.
11. Lary B: Postoperative suppurative parotitis. Arch Surg 89:653, 1964.
12. David R: Suppurative parotitis in children. Am J Dis Child 119:332, 1970.

13. Maxwell J: Chronic lymphoepithelial sialadenopathy with sialodochiectasis. Trans Amer Acad Ophthal Otolaryngol 64:225, 1960.
14. Shearn M: Sjögren's Syndrome. Philadelphia, W. B. Saunders Co., 1971.
15. Rausch S: Diseases of the salivary glands. In Gorlin R (ed): Thoma's Oral Pathology. Vol 2. 6th ed. St. Louis, C. V. Mosby, 1974, Chap 22.
16. Batsakis JG: Tumors of the Head and Neck. 2nd ed. Baltimore, Williams & Wilkins, 1979, p. 100.
17. Furstenberg AC, Blatt IM: Intermittent parotid swelling due to ill-fitting dentures - an entity, its diagnosis and treatment. Laryngoscope 68:1165, 1958.
18. Rausch S: Die Spiecheldruse Des Menchen. Stuttgart, Georg Thieme Verlag, 1959, p. 344.
19. Mandel ID, Baurmash H: Sialochemistry in chronic recurrent patotitis: electrolytes and glucose. J Oral Path 9:92, 1980.
20. Burgen ASV: Secretory processes in salivary glands. In Handbook of Physiology. Section 6, Vol 1. Washington DC, American Physiological Society, 1967, Chap 35.
21. Tobak L, Mandel ID, Kerlin D, Baurmash H: Alterations in lactoferrin in salivary gland disease. J Dent Res 67:43, 1978.
22. Casterline PF, Jaques DP: The surgical management of recurrent parotitis. Surg Gynecol Obstet 146:419, 1978.
23. Rankow RM, Polayes IM: Diseases of the Salivary Glands. Philadelphia, W. B. Saunders Company, 1976, Chap 9.
24. Batsakis JG, Bernacki EG, Rice DH, Stebler ME: Malignancy and the benign lymphoepithelial lesion. Laryngoscope 85:389, 1975.
25. Batsakis JG, Sylvest V: Pathology of the Salivary Glands. Chicago, American Society of Clinical Pathologists, 1977.
26. Batsakis JG: Tumors of the Head and Neck. 2nd ed. Baltimore, Williams & Wilkins Company, 1979, p. 106.
27. Fishback M, Char D, Christensen M, Daniels T, Whaley K, Alspaugh M, Talal N: Immune complexes in Sjögren's syndrome. Arthritis Rheum 23:791, 1980.
28. Arthaud JB: Anaplastic parotid carcinoma ("malignant lyphoepithelial lesions") in seven Alaskan natives. Am J Clin Pathol 24:744, 1971.
29. Chudwin DS, Daniels TE, Wara DW, Ammann AJ, Barrett DJ, Whitcher JP, Dowan MJ: Spectrum of Sjögren's syndrome in children. J Pediatr 98:213, 1981.
30. Shearn MA: Sjögren's syndrome. Med Clin N Amer 61:271, 1977.
31. Hadden WB: On "dry mouth" or suppression of the salivary and buccal secretions. Trans Clin Soc Lond 27:176, 1888.
32. Mikulicz J: Ueber eine eignartige symmetrische Erkankung der Thranen und Mundspeicheldrusen. Beitr Chir Festchrift Billroth 2:610, 1892.
33. Sjögren H: Zur kenntnis der keratoconjunctivitis sicca (Keratitis filiforms bei hypofunktion der tranendrusen). Acta Ophthalmol 11:1, 1933.
34. Morgan WS, Castleman B: A clinicopathologic study of Mikulicz's disease. Am J Path 29:471, 1953.
35. Moutsopoulos HM (Moderator): Sjögren's syndrome (sicca syndrome): current issues. Ann Intern Med 92:212, 1980.
36. Chused TM, Kassan SS, Opelz G, Moutsopoulos HM, Terasaki PI: Sjögren's syndrome associated with HLA-DW3. N Engl J Med 296:895, 1977.
37. Moutsopoulos HM, Mann DL, Johnson AH, Chused TM: Genetic differences between primary and secondary sicca syndrome. N Engl J Med 301:761, 1979.
38. Moutsopoulos HM, Webber BL, Vlagapoulos TP, Chused TM, Decker JL: Differences in the clinical manifestations of sicca syndrome in the presence and absence of rheumatoid arthritis. Am J Med 66:733, 1979.
39. Alspaugh MA, Talal N, Ton EM: Differentiation and characterization of autoantibodies and their antigens in Sjögren's syndrome. Arthritis Rheum 19:216, 1976.
40. Dawley T, Moutsopoulos HM, Katz SI, Theofilopoulos AN, Chused TM, Frank MM: Demonstration of circulating immune complexes in Sjögren's syndrome. J Immunol 123:1382, 1979.
41. Ichikawa Y, Takaya M, Arimori S: Cellular immunity to secretory IgA (as a common

duct antigen of exocrine glands) in Sjögren's syndrome. Tokai J Exp Clin Med 5:211, 1980.

42. Moutsopoulos HM, Fauci AS: Immunoregulation in Sjogren's syndrome: influence of serum factors on T-cell subpopulations. J Clin Invest 65:519, 1980.
43. Rubin P, Holt J: Secretory sialography in diseases of the major salivary glands. Am J Roentgen 77:575, 1957.
44. Som PM, Shugar JM, Train JS, Biller HF: Manifestations of parotid gland enlargement: radiographic pathologic, and clinical correlations. Part I. The autoimmune pseudosialectasias. Radiology 141:415, 1981.
45. Takeda Y: Histopathological studies of the labial salivary glands in patients with Sjögren's syndrome. Part II: electron microscopic study. Bull Tokyo Med Dent Univ 27:27, 1980.
46. Greenspan JS, Daniels TE, Talal N, Sylvester RA: The histopathology of Sjögren's syndrome in labial salivary gland biopsies. Oral Surg 32:217, 1974.
47. Moutsopoulos HM, Karsh J, Wolf RO, Tarpley TM, Tylenda A, Popodopoulos NM: Lysozyme determination in parotid saliva from patients with Sjögren's syndrome. Am J Med 69:39, 1980.
48. Avisar R, Menache R, Shaked P, Rubinstern J, Machtey I, Savir H: Lysozyme content of tears in patients with Sjögren's syndrome and rheumatoid arthritis. Am J Ophthalmol 87:148, 1979.
49. Mandel ID, Baurmash H: Sialochemistry in Sjögren's syndrome. Oral Surg Oral Med Oral Path 41:182, 1976.
50. Bertram U, Theilade J: Ultrastructural changes in the striated ducts of salivary glands of mice with autoimmune chronic sialadenitis. J. Dent Res 56:A87, 1977.
51. Tapper-John L, Aldred M, Walker DM: Prevalence and intraoral distribution of *Candida albicans* in Sjögren's syndrome. J. Clin Pathol 33:282, 1980.
52. Kassan SS, Thomas TL, Moutsopoulos HM et al.: Increased risk of lymphoma in sicca syndrome. Ann Intern Med 89:888, 1979.
53. Faguet GB, Webb HH, Agee JF, Richs WB, Sharbaugh AH: Immunologically diagnosed malignancy in Sjögren's pseudolymphoma. Am J Med 65:424, 1978.
54. Zulman J, Jaffee R, Talal N: Evidence that the malignant lymphoma of Sjögren's syndrome is a monoclonal B-cell neoplasm. N Engl J Med 299:1215, 1978.
55. MacGregor GA: Primary biliary cirrhosis in a dry-gland syndrome. Lancet 1:535, Sept. 6, 1980.
56. Vogel C, Wittenberg A, Reichart P: The involvement of the liver in Sjögren's syndrome. Oral Surg 50:26, 1980.
57. Prytz S: Vocal nodules in Sjögren's syndrome. J Laryngol Otol 94:197, 1980.
58. Barrs DM, McDonald TJ, Duffy J: Sjögren's syndrome involving the larynx: report of a case. J Laryngol Otol 93, 933, 1979.
59. Schwartzberg M, Burnstein SL, Calabro JJ, Jacobs JB: The development of membranous glomerulonphritis in a patient with rheumatoid arthritis and Sjögren's syndrome. J Rheumatol 6:65, 1979.
60. Fink AI, MacKay CJ, Cutler SS: Sicca complex and cholangiostatic jaundice in two members of a family probably caused by thiabendazole. Ophthalmology 86:1892, 1979.
61. Catalano MA, Vaughan JH: Secondary amyloidosis and sicca syndrome. Arthritis Rheum 23, 1067, 1980.
62. Pfister RR, Murphy GE: Corneal ulceration and perforation associated with Sjögren's syndrome. Arch Ophthalmol 98:89, 1980.
63. Horrabin DF, Campbell A: Sjögren's syndrome and the sicca syndrome: the role of prostaglandin E1 deficiency. Treatment with essential fatty acids and vitamin C. Med Hypothesis 6:225, 1980.
64. Cummings N, Schall L, Asofsky R, Talal N: Sjögren's syndrome. National Institutes of Health Conference. Ann Int Med 75:937, 1971.
65. Andersen L, Cummings N: Salivary gland immunoglobulin and rheumatoid factor synthesis in Sjögren's syndrome. Am J Med 53,456, 1972.
66. Esker BN: Obstructive inflammatory disease of the major salivary glands. Oral Surg 33:2, 1972.

67. Wong ML, Jafek BW: Cervical mycobacterial disease. Trans Am Acad Ophthal Otol 78:75, 1974.
68. Hammer JE, Goefield HH: Cervical lymphadenopathy and parotid gland swelling in sarcoidosis: a study of 31 cases. J Am Dent Assoc 74:1224, 1967.
69. Cahn L, Eisenbud L, Blake M, Stern D: Biopsy of normal appearing palates of patients with sarcoidosis. Oral Surg 18:342, 1964.
70. Turiaf J. Battesti JP: Gongerot-Sjögren's syndrome and sarcoidosis. Ann NY Acad Sci 28:401, 1976.
71. Batsakis, JG: Tumors of the Head and Neck. 2nd ed. Williams & Wilkins Company, Baltimore, 1979, pg 103.
72. Bhoola KD, McNichol NW, Oliver S, Foran J: Changes in salivary enzymes in patients with sarcoidosis. N Engl J Med 281:877, 1969.
73. Chisolm DM, Lyell A, Haroon TS, Mason DK, Beeley JA: Salivary gland function in sarcoidosis. Oral Surg Oral Med Oral Path 31:766, 1971.
74. Beeley, Chisolm DM: Sarcoidosis with salivary gland involvement: biochemical studies on parotid saliva. J Lab Clin Med 88:276, 1976.
75. Wagenvoort JH, Hansen M, Bentahar-Trouw BJ, Kraaijeveld CA, Windkler KC: Epidermiology of mumps in the Netherlands. J Hyg 85:313, 1980.
76. Freeman R, Hamblin MH: Serological studies in 40 cases of mumps virus infection. J Clin Pathol 33:28, 1980.
77. Helmke K, Otten A, Willems W: Islet cell antibodies in children with mumps infection. Lancet 2:221, 1980.
78. Gamble DR: Relation to antecedent illness to development of diabetes in children. Br Med J 281:99, 1980.

Chapter Four

NONINFLAMMATORY, NON-NEOPLASTIC DISORDERS

SIALOLITHIASIS

Eighty per cent of salivary calculi occur in the submandibular gland, whereas less than 20 per cent occur in the parotid, and 1 per cent occur in the sublingual gland. Minor salivary gland calculi are uncommon and have a predilection for the upper lip and buccal mucosa.[1] They are usually asymptomatic, freely mobile, and less than 0.5 cm in diameter. For the major glands, there is a single calculus in 75 per cent of cases and multiple gland involvement in 3 per cent. They usually occur in middle age and there is a slight male predominance. Calculi may occur unassociated with other salivary disease, but also occur in two-thirds of cases of chronic sialadenitis. The majority of calculi are composed largely of calcium phosphate as the hydroxyapatite and small amounts of magnesium, carbonate, and ammonium. The organic matrix is composed of various carbohydrates and amino acids. Ninety per cent of submandibular calculi are radiopaque, but 90 percent of parotid calculi are radiolucent. Prerequisites for calculus formation are stasis and a nidus of material for the precipitation of salivary salts. There is some evidence that most submandibular calculi arise de novo around a nidus of mucus, whereas parotid calculi are preceded by an inflammatory response and form around inflammatory cells.[2] This difference is uncertain at present. The submandibular gland is believed to be more susceptible because its saliva is more alkaline, has a greater concentration of calcium and phosphate,[3] and has a higher mucus content. In addition, the duct is longer, and the flow is antigravity. The only systemic disease associated with salivary calculi is gout, and the calculi are then composed of uric acid.

Occasionally calculi are asymptomatic or appear as acute suppurative sialadenitis. More commonly the patient gives a history of recurrent swelling and pain in the involved gland, usually associated with eating. With repeated episodes, infection may intervene. In general, sialoliths within the glandular parenchyma are associated with less severe symptoms than those producing obstruction of the main duct. Physical examination reveals diffuse enlargement and tenderness of the involved gland. The calculus is frequently palpable. Calculi within the duct tend to be smooth, but those within the gland tend to be irregular. Massage of the gland demonstrates decreased flow of cloudy, perhaps mucopurulent, saliva. For the usual submandibular gland radiopaque calculus, routine mandibular roentgenograms suffice for the diagnosis. For parotid calculi, an anteroposterior roentgenogram coupled with an intrabuccal film reveal a calculus 71 per cent of the time.[4] For either gland, sialography is essentially 100 per cent effective. Untrasound also may be used.[5]

Complications of sialolithiasis include acute suppurative sialadenitis and ductal ulceration and stricture. Treatment depends on the location of the calculus. If it is near the duct orifice, intraoral removal is simple and curative. After establishing adequate local anesthesia, a probe is inserted into the duct to the calculus. The duct is then incised over the probe until the calculus is reached, and the calculus can then be extracted. Repair of the duct is not necessary. If the calculus is within the hilum of the submandibular gland, complete excision of the gland is curative and is performed if symptoms are unacceptable or if frequent infections occur. For the parotid gland also, an attempt at conservative therapy is prudent. However, if recurrent infections occur, a parotidectomy should be performed. In situations in which only the calculus is removed, the recurrence rate may be as high as 18 per cent,[6] since the underlying cause, which is unknown, has not been corrected.

On rare occasions a calcified phlebolith may be mistaken radiographically for an asymptomatic salivary calculus. Several differences help to separate them. Phleboliths are usually circular, laminated, and multiple. On sialography they are outside the duct system.[7,8]

CYSTIC LESIONS

True cysts of salivary tissue are unusual and the majority occur in the parotid, where they account for 2 to 5 per cent of all parotid lesions. Cysts may be acquired or congenital, and there are three types of congenital cysts. The *dermoid cyst,* which consists of keratinizing squamous epithelium with associated skin appendages, is treated by complete removal with preservation of the facial nerve. The *congenital ductal cyst* is generally manifest in infancy. The diagnosis generally requires sialography under general anesthesia. No therapy is required unless repeated infections occur.[9] The *first arch branchial groove cyst* accounts for less that 1 per cent of all branchial arch anomalies. There are two distinct first groove anomalies, classified as type I and type II (Figure 4–1). Type I is ectodermal and a lesion of the first cleft only. Type II is ectodermal and mesodermal and is a lesion of the first and second arches.[10] The former is a duplication anomaly of the membranous external auditory canal, the latter a duplication

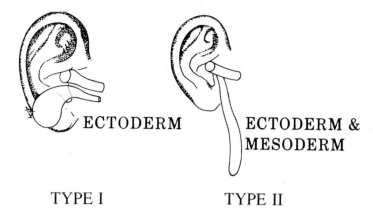

ECTODERM

ECTODERM &
MESODERM

TYPE I

TYPE II

Figure 4–1. Type I and Type II first arch branchial cleft cysts.

anomaly of the membranous and cartilaginous external auditory canal. The type I cyst typically occurs posterior, inferior, or anterior to the ear, and may bear any relationship to the facial nerve. Prior infection, with and without incision and drainage, may mask the true nature of the lesion. Complete excision during a quiescent period, with preservation of the facial nerve, is curative. The type II lesion may occur from the preauricular area to the hyoid bone. Regardless of the location, the tract is intimately associated with the facial nerve. Again, frequent prior infections may obscure the true lesion. Excision during a quiescent period, with preservation of the facial nerve, is curative.

Acquired cysts may be secondary to neoplasms, the benign lymphoepithelial lesion, trauma, parotitis, calculi, duct obstruction, and mucus extravasation.[11] The presence of a cystic lesion does not preclude the possibility of a neoplasm, especially the pleomorphic adenoma, the adenoid cystic carcinoma, the mucoepidermoid carcinoma, and Warthin's tumor.[8] These are the neoplasms most commonly cystic and are also the most common salivary gland neoplasms. When appropriate, for the other acquired cysts, the underlying cause should be treated first. If that fails, or if the cyst becomes repeatedly infected, excision should be performed. This would include the rare epidermoid cyst and the rare lymphoepithelial cyst.[12] Mucoceles and mucus retention cysts usually involve the minor salivary glands and most commonly occur in the lips, cheeks, and ventral tongue. Mucus retention cysts are true cysts with an epithelial lining and result from partial duct obstruction. Complete duct obstruction leads to glandular atrophy.[13,14] Mucoceles do not possess an epithelial lining and are not true cysts. Instead they represent mucus extravasation into the soft tissues. Treatment is by excision or marsupialization if treatment is required. Propantheline bromide has been recommended as a trial treatment in sialoceles that involve the parotid so as to avoid parotidectomy.[15] The simple ranula is a mucus retention cyst of the sublingual gland.[8] The so-called plunging ranula is a mucocele that extends from the floor of the mouth into the neck. The treatment is excision.[16]

TRAUMA

Direct injuries of note usually involve a penetrating injury that lacerates the duct. Any penetrating injury to the cheek posterior to the anterior border of the masseter muscle should be suspected of causing a duct injury. Inspection of the wound often reveals the status of the duct. If the duct cannot be identified, a probe may be passed into the duct transorally and located in the wound. This should confirm the status of the duct. If the duct has been transected, the optimum treatment is immediate end-to-end anastomosis over a polyethylene catheter with 9-0 sutures. The catheter is sutured in place to the buccal mucosa and removed in 2 weeks. If the proximal end of the duct cannot be readily identified, the following maneuver may help: The wound should be made as dry as possible; compression of the gland then often produces enough saliva from the cut end of the duct to allow its identification. If primary anastomosis is impossible, but the proximal duct is long enough, the duct may be sutured directly to the buccal mucosa through a puncture wound. If the proximal duct is too short, several choices are available. The duct may be ligated. This will usually lead to atrophy of the gland, although infection or a salivary-cutaneous fistula may result. The second choice is to construct a new distal duct from buccal mucosa.[17] In all these situations, repeated dilatation with lacrimal probes may be necessary to achieve a satisfactory final result.[18]

Occasionally a duct injury is missed only to become manifest several days later as a swelling below the sutured wound. In this situation, the wound must be opened and the duct identified and repaired.

Laceration of the parenchyma, in isolation, can usually be managed conservatively. Generally, merely closing the parenchyma and capsule with a few interrupted sutures will suffice. Occasionally a salivary-cutaneous fistula develops, but can be healed by repeated aspiration and a pressure dressing. Resolution often takes 7 to 14 days, by which time the traumatized ductal system will have re-opened. Persistence of a fistula strongly suggests duct obstruction rather than parenchymal injury alone.[19] Sialography should be performed to investigate this. If ductal obstruction is found, repair should be performed if possible. If repair of the duct is impossible and the fistula persists, a tympanic neurectomy may help.[20] Occasionally a salivary-cutaneous fistula can be diverted into the oral cavity. The entire fistulous tract is excised, turned into the oral cavity through the cheek, and sutured to the buccal mucosa.[21] If that fails, excision of the gland or irradiation to destroy the gland is carried out. Irradiation is probably ill-advised in the younger patient. Sometimes a sialocele develops instead of a fistula, and it may occur in the absence of penetrating trauma.[22]

Penetrating injuries can also transect one or more branches of the facial nerve. A thorough evaluation of the facial nerve should be performed on any patient who has suffered a penetrating injury to the face. If the wound is anterior to a vertical line from the lateral canthus to the mental foramen (a line approximating the anterior border of the masseter muscle) and only a single branch is involved, repair is probably unnecessary. In this instance recovery is likely from distal anastomosing branches. Posterior to this line, repair should be performed immediately (see the section on facial nerve injury in this chapter).

Besides penetrating injury, duct strictures can be caused by calculi, infection, blunt trauma, and neoplasms. Congenital strictures also occur. Duct strictures present with periodic swelling and tenderness, usually associated with eating. Intermittent infection may occur. A sialogram is diagnostic, and management depends on the cause. If the underlying problem is identifiable and treatable, attention should be first directed toward this problem. If the stricture persists, periodic dilatation should be performed. If that fails and the stricutre is near the natural orifice, a sialodochoplasty should be performed. If that is not possible or if it fails and symptoms continue to be significant, excision of the gland should be performed.

Blunt trauma can also injure the gland causing contusions, edema, or hemorrhage. Contusions and edema usually resolve without treatment, although temporary duct obstruction may occur. A hematoma, if significant, should be drained before it becomes organized. If not, subsequent fibrosis and scarring may lead to duct obstruction as well as to cosmetic deformity.

In general, injury to the submandibular or sublingual glands are managed in the same way as injury to the parotid. Penetrating injuries other than parenchymal laceration are uncommon because of the protection afforded by the mandible. If the injury does not heal satisfactorily, excision of the gland should be performed.

RADIATION INJURY

Salivary glands may undergo irradiation damage for several reasons— as the primary target for chronic infection or neoplasm or as a secondary effect while irradiation is being directed at some other neoplasm. Low-dose irradiation causes an acute, tender, painful swelling of salivary tissue.

The serous cells and acini are exquisitely sensitive and exhibit marked degranulation and disruption, which cause pools of zymogen granules to appear in the acini. Simultaneously an acute inflammatory reaction causes a purulent exudate within the ducts as well as parenchymal suppuration. In contrast the mucous cells and acini, and the epithelial cells of the intercalated and interlobular ducts exhibit little histologic change. The acute inflammatory reaction subsides without treatment, provided the irradiation is stopped. Continued irradiation leads to complete destruction of the serous acini and subsequent atrophy of the gland. See Chapter 1 for more complete discussion of the effects of irradiation upon salivary glands.

Radiation-induced thyroid neoplasms are well documented, and there is growing evidence that salivary and parathyroid tumors are also induced.[23-26] A significant increase in malignant neoplasms when compared to nonirradiated controls has been reported.[27] Multiple carcinomas have been reported.[28] The parotid gland is the most common site of neoplasia, and mucoepidermoid carcinoma is the most common malignant neoplasm. An increased risk of developing a pleomorphic adenoma has also been reported.[29]

SIALADENOSIS

Sialadenosis is a nonspecific term used to describe a noninflammatory, non-neoplastic enlargement of a salivary gland, usually the parotid. There are many causes of sialadenosis (Table 4–1), the mechanism being generally unknown. The salivary gland enlargement is usually asymptomatic.

Bilateral parotid swelling is common in obesity. A complete endocrinologic and metabolic work-up should be performed before the diagnosis of fatty hypertrophy is made. This is because obesity is frequently associated with other disorders such as diabetes mellitus, hypertension, hyperlipidemia, and menopause. In particular, hypertrophy is frequently associated with diabetes mellitus and has been reported in acromegaly.

Malnutrition is frequently associated with sialadenosis, but it is also associated with pellagra, cirrhosis, diabetes mellitus, and beriberi.[30] In these people the level of proteinemia is usually from 3 to 6 gm per cent.[31] Sialadenosis has been reported in kwashiorkor (literally, red boy) and hypovitaminosis A. The swelling in these conditions is due to acinar hypertrophy.

The association of parotid swelling with alcoholic cirrhosis is well recognized. It is so rare in nonalcoholic cirrhosis that it can be used as a differential diagnostic feature.[32] In alcoholic cirrhosis, parotid enlargement occurs in 30 to 80 per cent of cases. Current evidence suggests that

TABLE 4–1 Non-Neoplastic, Noninflammatory Causes of Salivary Enlargement

I. Nutritional Deficiency
  A. Hypoproteinemia
  B. Pellegra
  C. Beriberi
  D. Hypovitaminosis A
  E. Generalized malnutrition
  F. Obesity
II. Metabolic or Endocrine Abnormalities
  A. Any malabsorption disorder
  B. Pregnancy
  C. Lactation
  D. Menopause
  E. Diabetes mellitus
  F. Hypothyroidism
  G. Testicular atrophy
  H. Uremia
  I. Alcoholic cirrhosis
III. Other
  A. Drugs
  B. Pneumoparotitis
  C. Kussmaul's disease

the enlargement is based on protein deficiency, and the histologic changes are similar to those in malnutrition. In these patients, the salivary output is normal, but the amylase is increased.

As already implied, any disease that disrupts gastrointestinal absorption of nutrients may lead to parotid hypertrophy. Reported diseases include celiac disease, bacillary dysentery, carcinoma of the esophagus, Chagas' disease, and ancylostomiasis.[33] Sialadenosis may also occur in uremia, hypothyroidism, myxedema, testicular or ovarian atrophy, pregnancy, lactation, and chronic relapsing pancreatitis.

The prognosis of sialadenosis is generally good. The parotid glands usually revert to normal following correction of the underlying cause.

OTHER NONINFLAMMATORY, NON-NEOPLASTIC DISORDERS

A number of drugs may cause salivary enlargement as a side-effect. Thiourea, isoproterenol, methimazole, phenylbutazone, phenothiazine, thiocyanate, iodine compounds, and the heavy metals have been implicated. See Chapter 1 for a more complete discussion.

Pneumoparotitis may result from any factor that increases intrabuccal pressure. It has been reported in glass blowers, following intubation or endoscopy, and as an idiopathic event.[34]

Kussmaul's disease (sialodochitis fibrinosis) consists of a mucous plug obstructing a collecting duct. This usually occurs in a dehydrated patient and is manifest by recurrent swelling with associated pain. The appearance of a mucous plug at the duct orifice is diagnostic. Treatment consists of gentle massage and sialogogues to extrude the plug, in addition to rehydration where appropriate.

Occasionally attention is directed to the salivary glands because of uncontrolled drooling. This generally occurs in the neurologically damaged child or adult. A number of treatments have been advocated to correct or ameliorate this problem. Good results have been reported with bilateral tympanic neurectomy as well as in submandibular duct relocation.[35,36] Satisfactory results have been reported with parotid duct relocation.[37] A more aggressive approach has advocated bilateral parotid duct relocation combined with bilateral submandibular gland excision.[38] In general, drooling should be treated in a progressive manner, with each additional procedure indicated only by failure of the preceding procedure.

Radiation should be reserved for operative failures to avoid the side-effects of xerostomia and increased dental caries, which can be significant management problems in themselves in these patients. Further it should be used only in adults to reduce the risk of induced malignancy. One interesting approach that has met with some success has involved training the patient to swallow in response to an auditory clue emanating from a small noise maker pinned to the patient's clothes.[39]

Cheilitis glandularis is an uncommon disease characterized by enlarged labial salivary glands, which secrete a clear, thick, sticky mucus.[40] The glandular hypertrophy may cause eversion of the lower lip. Vermilionectomy is generally curative.

Necrotizing sialometoplasia is a disease of cryptogenic etiology, although some cases appear to occur as a reaction to injury. It generally begins as a mucosal ulceration in the hard palate, but may occur anywhere salivary tissue is found, including the nasopharynx.[41] There is a male predominance. It was first reported in 1973,[42] and its importance lies in the fact that it can be mistaken for squamous cell or mucoepidermoid carcinoma. Histologically there is mucosal ulceration with pseudoepitheliomatous hyperplasia, ischemic lobular necrosis, dissolution of acinar walls with the release of mucus which causes a subsequent inflammatory and granulation tissue response, and squamous metaplasia of acini and ducts. As of 1980, there had been 40 cases reported.[43] The lesion is always self-healing and requires no treatment other than biopsy.

Aberrant salivary tissue can occur in a variety of locations. It is not unusual to find aberrant salivary tissue within lymph nodes, especially in the parotid area. It has been reported in 1 per cent of tonsils. Salivary tissue has been reported in the mandible, lower neck, hypopharynx, middle ear, sternoclavicular joint, thyroglossal duct, and pituitary gland.[44] In the mandible, the tissue may be on the surface or central. Those on the surface appear to be merely ectopic submandibular tissue and are always benign. Central lesions are uncommon and even less common in the maxilla. When these tissues become neoplastic, the type of tumor may be mucoepidermoid carcinoma, adenoid cystic carcinoma, or adenocarcinoma, in descending order of frequency.[45]

MANAGEMENT OF FACIAL PARALYSIS

The facial nerve can be damaged in a variety of ways within the parotid gland, but the most common causes of damage are malignant neoplasms, parotid surgery, and penetrating trauma. Optimal rehabilitation depends on the extent, location, and duration of the injury (Figure 4–2).

The ideal repair for a transection of either a branch or the main trunk of the facial nerve is immediate end-to-end anastomosis. Although some believe that there is a theoretical advantage to delay of the repair,[46] the distal nerve can be difficult or impossible to identify once it loses its ability to respond to electrical stimulation. Further, recent studies suggest that primary repair is superior to delayed repair.[47,48] The duration of stimulability is generally 3 days, but may be lost in less than 48 hours. For this reason, any patient with an acute penetrating injury to the region of the parotid gland who has a partial or total facial paralysis should be taken immediately to the operating room for exploration and repair. The exception to this is the patient with multiple injuries who is not stable, in which case, if it is possible, the wound should be rapidly explored and the ends of the nerve identified and tagged. Repair can then be accomplished when the patient is able to undergo repair in the operating room.

Similarly, the main trunk of the facial nerve should be stimulated just prior to closure after a parotidectomy. If any region of the face fails to move, the branch to that region should be carefully explored. If the nerve has been transected, immediate repair should be performed. One should never assume that the nerve is intact and close without exploring the branch in question.

There are several methods of repair advocated for end-to-end anastomosis: (1) epineural repair[49] (Figure 4–3); (2) fascicular repair[50] (Figure 4–4); and (3) fascicular repair with the amount of suture material used kept at a minimum.[51] Clearly the minimum suture material used would follow epineural repair. Reported results are similar. A recent randomized prospective comparison found no difference.[52]

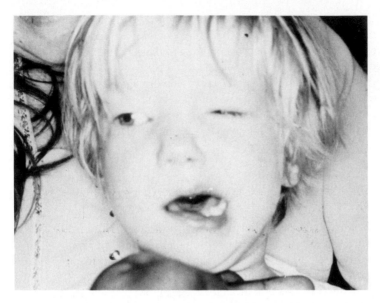

Figure 4–2. An example of facial nerve paralysis secondary to a single bite by the family St. Bernard. Note the facial asymmetry while crying.

If a portion of the nerve has been resected during parotidectomy or traumatically avulsed, the ideal repair is a cable graft, performed immediately so that the distal nerve can be identified. Cable grafts, which were first used in 1870,[53] should be used even if one must enter the temporal bone to reach the proximal stump. Repair can be accomplished as far medially as the cerebellopontine angle.[54] Any nerve of appropriate size, length, and branching pattern may be used for this graft, but the two most commonly used are the great auricular and the lateral femoral cutaneous nerves.

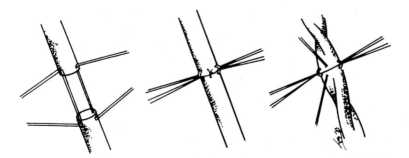

Figure 4–3. Epineural repair. Modified from Miehlke A: Surgery of the Facial Nerve, W. B. Saunders Company, Philadelphia, 1973.

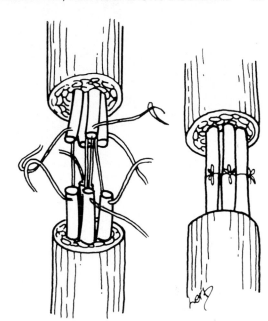

Figure 4–4. Fascicular repair. Modified from Miehlke A: Surgery of the Facial Nerve, W. B. Saunders Company, Philadelphia, 1973.

If for some reason the proximal facial nerve is unavailable for repair, other techniques may prove useful. If the injury is in the parotid gland, however, the need for other techniques should be quite rare. The most popular of these techniques involves using the proximal portion of another motor nerve for anastomosis to the distal branch of the facial nerve. The accessory nerve was first used in 1879[55] and then in 1900,[56] and the hypoglossal and glossopharyngeal nerves in 1924.[57] The hypoglossal is currently preferred. These repairs are unphysiologic and decidedly inferior to direct repair of the facial nerve. However, they will supply good facial tone and some motion. Some patients, after considerable practice, can develop excellent voluntary motion. These repairs do not restore appropriate facial motion in response to emotional stimuli.[50]

The proximal facial nerve is almost always available in cases of parotid disease. However, the distal branches may not be, especially if the patient is seen some time after the injury and the distal branch cannot be identified or if the distal branch has been resected during removal of a malignant neoplasm. Rehabilitation in this situation is much less satisfactory, but can still be beneficial.

Although several techniques are available, the most popular technique involves the temporalis and masseter muscles (Figure 4–5). Part of the superior portion of the temporalis muscle is dissected free as an inferiorly based pedicle flap. It is turned over and sutured into the orbicularis oculi

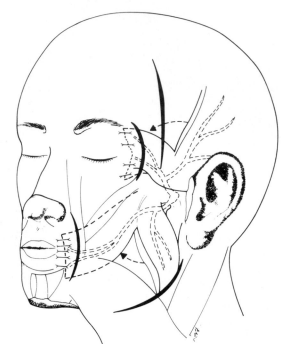

Figure 4–5. The temporalis and masseter muscles used to support the face. Modified from Miehlke A: Surgery of the Facial Nerve, W. B. Saunders Company, Philadelphia, 1973.

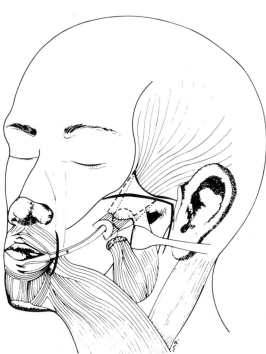

Figure 4–6. An appoplast used to support the face. Modified from Miehlke A: Surgery of the Facial Nerve, W. B. Saunders Company, Philadelphia, 1973.

muscle. In addition, a superiorly based pedicle flap of the masseter muscle is sutured into the orbicularis oris muscle. It was once thought that several nerve endings in the pedicled muscle would migrate into the recepient muscle and reinnervate it. Experimental evidence strongly indicates that this does not occur.[50] For these techniques to work, the motor division of the trigeminal nerve must be intact.

Another technique involves the use of an alloplast as a sling. The most commonly used materials are nylon, Tantalum, and Marlex (Figure 4–6). The slings may be placed as static supports or may be attached superiorly to the temporalis muscle pedicle.

A third technique, introduced to reinnervate the corner of the mouth, involves using a nerve-muscle pedicle from the ansa cervicalis.[58] Transected nerve endings are supposed to grow into the orbicularis oris and reinnervate it. As mentioned, experimental evidence argues against this.

For a time, cable grafts from the contralateral facial nerve to the distal branches of the injured facial nerve held some popularity. The test of time has been disappointing with this technique and it is no longer advised.[59]

When the branches to the eye are involved and the patient is awaiting return of function, a tarsorrhaphy may be necessary. Absence of the normal blink and incomplete closure at night expose the cornea to desiccation. If the irritation is not severe enough to require a tarsorrhaphy, the use of artificial tears during the day and taping the lids closed at night may suffice.

Electromyography may be useful in following the results of nerve repair, as it can demonstrate the presence of reinnervation before it is clinically apparent. Denervated muscle is irritable and shows fibrillation potentials at rest and no motor unit action potentials on attempted motion. During recovery, electromyography shows the development of motor unit action potentials and decrease in fibrillation potentials several weeks before motion is clinically detectable.

REFERENCES

1. Jensen JL, Howell FV, Rick, GM, Correll RW: Minor salivary gland calculi. A clinicopathologic study of forty-seven new cases. Oral Surg 47:44, 1979.
2. Mason DK, Chisolm DM: Salivary Glands in Health and Disease. Philadelphia, W. B. Saunders, 1975.
3. Blatt IM: Studies in sialolithiasis. III. Pathogenesis, diagnosis, and treatment. South Med J 57:733, 1964.
4. Suleiman SI, Hobsley M: Radiological appearances of parotid duct calculi. Br J Surg 67:879, 1980.
5. Pickerell KL, Trought WS, Shearin JC: The use of ultrasound to localize calculi within the parotid gland. Ann Plast Surg 1:542, 1978.
6. Levy, Remine W, Devine K: Salivary gland calculi. JAMA 181:1115, 1962.
7. O'Riordan B: Phleboliths and salivary calculi. Br J Oral Surg 12:119, 1974.

8. Anneroth G, Eneroth DM, Isaccson G: Angiolithiasis in the parotid gland. Int J Oral Surg 7:1139, 1978.
9. Work WP: Cysts and congenital lesions of the parotid gland. Otolaryngol Clin N Amer 10:339, 1977.
10. Aronsohn RS, Batsakis JG, Rice DH, Work WP: Anomalies of the first branchial cleft. Arch Otolaryngol 102:737, 1976.
11. Work WP, Hecht DW: Non-neoplastic lesions of the parotid gland. Ann Otol Rhinol Laryngol 77:462, 1968.
12. Bernier JL, Bhaskar SN: Lymphoepithelial lesions of salivary glands. Cancer 11:1156, 1958.
13. Batsakis JG: Tumors of the Head and Neck. Baltimore, Williams & Wilkins, 1979, p. 117.
14. Sela J, Ulmansky M: Mucus retention cyst of salivary glands. J Oral Surg 27:619, 1969.
15. Krausen AS, Ogura JH: Sialoceles: medical treatment first. Trans Am Acad Opthalmol Otolaryngol 84:890, 1977.
16. Quick CA, Lowell SH: Ranula and the sublingual salivary glands. Arch Otolaryngol 103:397, 1977.
17. Padgett EC, Stephenson KL: Plastic and Reconstructive Surgery. Springfield, Ill, Charles C Thomas, 1947.
18. Olson NR: Traumatic lesions of the salivary glands. Otolaryngol Clin N Am 10:345, 1977.
19. Hemenway WG: Parotid duct fistula, a review. South Med J 64:912, 1971.
20. Chadwick SJ:, Davis WE, Templer JW: Parotid fistula: current management. South Med J 72:922, 1979.
21. Morel AS, Firestein A: Repair of traumatic fistulas of the parotid duct. Arch Surg 87:623, 1963.
22. Solomon AR, McClatchey KD, Batsakis JG: Serous extravasation granuloma. A parotid mass. Arch Otolaryngol 107:294, 1981.
23. Rice DH, Batsakis JG, McClatchey KD: Postirradiation malignant salivary gland tumor. Arch Otolaryngol 102, 699, 1976.
24. Schneider AB, Favus MJ, Stachura ME, Arnold MS, Frohman LA: Salivary gland neoplasms as a late consequence of head and neck irradiation. Ann Int Med 87:160, 1977.
25. Southwick HW: Radiation-associated head and neck tumors. Am J Surg 134:438, 1977.
26. Takeichi N, Hirose F, Yamamoto H: Salivary gland tumors in atomic bomb survivors. Cancer 38:2462, 1976.
27. Maxon HR, Saenger EL, Thomas SR, Shafer ML, Buncher CR, Kereiakes JG, McLaughlin CA: Radiation-associated carcinoma of the salivary glands. A controlled study. Ann Otol Rhinol Laryngol 90:107, 1981.
28. Senes SF, Scanlon EF: Irradiation induced salivary gland neoplasia. Ann Surg 191:304, 1980.
29. Batsakis JG: Tumors of the Head and Neck. 2nd ed. Baltimore, Williams & Wilkins, 1979, p. 16.
30. Keneway MR: Endemic enlargement of the parotid gland in Egypt. Trans R Soc Trip Med Hyg 31:339, 1937.
31. Yoel J: Pathology and Surgery of the Salivary Glands. Springfield, Ill, Charles C Thomas, 1975, p. 321.
32. Borsanyi SJ, Blanchard CL: Asymptomatic enlargement of the parotid glands: its diagnostic significance and particular relation to Laennec's cirrhosis. JAMA 174:20, 1960.
33. Gill G: Metabolic and endocrine influences on the salivary glands. Otolaryngol Clin N Amer 10:363, 1977.
34. Sarr MG, Frey H: A unique case of benign postoperative parotid swelling. Johns Hopkins Med J 146:11, 1980.
35. Crysdale WS: The drooling patient: evaluation and current surgical options. Laryngoscope 90:775, 1980.
36. Mullins WM, Gross CW, Moore JM: Long term follow-up of tympanic neurectomy for sialorrhea. Laryngoscope 89:1219, 1979.

37. Massengill R Jr: A follow-up investigation of patients who have had parotid duct transplantation surgery to control drooling. Ann Plast Surg 2:205, 1979.
38. Chait LA, Kessler E: An anti-drooling operation in cerebral palsy. S Afr Med J 56:676, 1979.
39. Rapp DL, Bowers PM: Meldreth dribble-control project. Child Care Health Dev 5:143, 1979.
40. Oliver ID, Pickett AB: Cheilitis glandularis. Oral Surg 49:526, 1980.
41. Merwin GE, Duckert LG, Pollak K: Necrotizing sialometaplasia of the nasopharynx. Ann Otol Rhinol Laryngol 88:348, 1979.
42. Abrams AM, Melrose RJ, Howell FV: Necrotizing sialometaplasia: a disease simulating malignancy. Cancer 32:130, 1973.
43. Gad A, Willen H, Willen R, Thorstensson S, Ekman L; Necrotizing sialometaplasia of the lip simulating squamous cell carcinoma. Histopathology 4:111, 1980.
44. Schocket SS, McCormick WF, Halmi NS: Salivary gland rests in the human pituitary. Light and electron microscopical study. Arch Path 98, 192, 1974.
45. Dhawan IK, Bhargova S, Nayak NC, Gupta RK: Central salivary gland tumors of jaws. Cancer 26:211, 1970.
46. Duker TB, Kempe LG, Hayes GJ: The metabolic background for peripheral nerve study. J Neurosurg 30:270, 1968.
47. Grabb WC: Median and ulner nerve suture. An experimental study comparing primary and secondary repair in monkeys. J Bone Joint Surg 50A:964, 1968.
48. Hatano E: A comparative study on primary and secondary nerve repair. Plast Reconstr Surg 68:760, 1981.
49. Conley J, Baker DC: The surgical treatment of extratemporal facial paralysis: an overview. Head Neck Surg 1:12, 1978.
50. Miehlke A: Surgery of the Facial Nerve. Philadelphia, W. B. Saunders Company, 1973.
51. Millesi H, Berger A, Meissl G: Experimentelle untersuchungen zur heilung durchtrennter peripherer nerven. Chir Plastica (Berlin) 1:174, 1972.
52. Young L, Wray RC, Weeks PM: A randomized prospective comparison of fascicular and epineural digital nerve repairs. Plastic Reconstr Surg 68:89, 1981.
53. Philipeaux and Vulpian, cited in Miehlke A: Surgery of the Facial Nerve. Philadelphia, W. B. Saunders Company, 1973, p. 3.
54. Brackmann D, Hitselberger W, Robinson J: Facial nerve repair in cerebellopontine angle surgery. Ann Otol Rhinol Laryngol 87:772, 1978.
55. Drobnik, cited in Miehlke A: Surgery of the Facial Nerve. Philadelphia, W. B. Saunders Company, 1973, p. 4.
56. Monasse P: Uber vereinigung des n. facialis mit dem. n. accessorius durch dire nervenpfropfung (graffe nerveuse). Arch Klin Chir 62:805, 1900.
57. Ballance C: Results obtained in some experiments in which the facial and recurrent nerves were anastomosed with other nerves. Br Med J 2:349, 1924.
58. Tucker HM: Restoration of selective facial nerve function by the nerve-muscle pedicle technique. Clin Plast Surg 6:293, 1979.
59. Crumley RL: Recent advances in facial nerve surgery. Head Neck Surg 4:233, 1982.

Chapter Five

BENIGN NEOPLASMS

Salivary gland neoplasms are uncommon and comprise less than 3 percent of all tumors.[1] Despite this, probably no organ system in the body produces such a large variety of neoplasms.[2] Seventh-five to 85 percent occur in the parotid, whereas 10 to 20 percent arise in the minor salivary glands, most commonly in the palate and tongue. An approximate incidence ratio is as follows: for every 100 parotid tumors, there are 10 submandibular gland tumors, 10 minor salivary gland tumors, and 1 sublingual tumor.[3] The relative incidence of malignant neoplasms increases as the size of the salivary gland decreases, except for the sublingual gland, which has the highest ratio of malignant to benign neoplasms. Eighty per cent of parotid, 65 percent of submandibular, 50 percent of minor salivary gland, and 20 percent of sublingual gland tumors are benign.[4,5]

The incidence and distribution of salivary gland tumors in white populations is essentially the same worldwide. African blacks have an increased incidence of pleomorphic adenomas in the minor and lesser major salivary glands.[6] Submandibular tumors occur with increased frequency among the Chinese in Malaya, the Africans in Uganda, and the West Indians. There is no significant sex distribution in whites, but nonwhite women have an increased incidence over nonwhite men.

In general, benign salivary gland tumors appear as an asymptomatic mass below intact skin or mucosa. The rate of growth is variable as is the duration of the mass. Since tumors of the parotid dominate the statistics, several additional generalizations can be made. Eighty per cent of parotid tumors arise in the caudal aspect of the superficial lobe. Thus every subcutaneous mass in the region of the inferior attachment of the ear should be considered a probable parotid neoplasm. Here as for benign tumors elsewhere, symptoms are usually absent, and the growth rate and duration of the mass are variable. Pain does not necessarily signify malignancy, as 5 per cent of benign and 6 per cent of malignant salivary neoplasms are painful when discovered. Deep lobe tumors may also appear as a mass at the angle of the mandible or as a parapharyngeal mass. In this setting, the facial nerve may be displaced laterally into a vulnerable position and may be damaged if the true situation is not recognized. The general treatment approach for benign tumors is complete excision. For the parotid, this

89

TABLE 5–1 Histogenesis of Salivary Gland Tumors

	Benign	*Malignant*
Intercalated duct reserve cell	Papillary adenoma Pleomorphic adenoma Monomorphic adenomas	Adenoid cystic carcinoma Acinous cell carcinoma
Excretory duct reserve cell	Intraductal papilloma	Squamous cell carcinoma Mucoepidermoid carcinoma Adenocarcinoma
Uncertain	Warthin's tumor Oncocytoma	

TABLE 5–2 Classification of Salivary Epithelial Neoplasms

Benign	Pleomorphic adenoma (benign mixed tumor)
	Papillary cystadenoma lymphomatosum (Warthin's tumor)
	Oncocytoma
	Monomorphic adenomas
	   Basal cell adenoma
	   Glycogen-rich adenoma
	   Membranous adenoma
	   Myoepithelioma
	Sebaceous tumors
	   Adenoma
	   Lymphadenoma
	Papillary ductal adenoma

Malignant	Mucoepidermoid carcinoma
	   Low-grade
	   Intermediate-grade
	   High-grade
	Adenoid cystic carcinoma
	Acinous cell carcinoma
	Adenocarcinoma
	   Mucus-producing adenocarcinomas
	   Salivary duct carcinoma
	   Other adenocarcinomas
	Carcinoma ex pleomorphic adenoma
	Malignant mixed tumor
	Oncocytic carcinoma
	Clear cell carcinoma
	Squamous cell carcinoma
	Hybrid basal cell adenoma/adenoid
	   cystic carcinoma
	Epithelial-myoepithelia carcinoma of intercalated ducts
	Miscellaneous carcinomas

means parotidectomy with preservation of the facial nerve. The facial nerve should never be sacrificed during excision of a benign tumor, except for the rare recurrent pleomorphic adenoma wherein tumor, scar, and nerve are so intimately intertwined that complete excision is impossible without sacrifice of the nerve. In this situation, consideration should be given to irradiation rather than operation. If part or all of the facial nerve is resected, immediate repair should be performed.

The histogenesis of salivary gland neoplasms has been considerably elucidated over the past decade. It is now generally agreed, as first pointed out in 1971,[7] that the basal cells of the excretory and intercalated ducts act as reserve cells for the more differentiated cells of the salivary gland unit. To the light microscopic evidence can now be added data from electron microscopic studies which further support the theory that all salivary gland epithelial neoplasms arise from these two cells—the excretory duct reserve cell and the intercalated duct reserve cell—and not by dedifferentiation of their mature counterparts.[8]

Thus neoplasia is the result of disease of the reserve cells, which are responsible for tissue renewal, and not of the fully differentiated cells.[9] The genome of these cells contains all the information needed to undergo normal development or to become a benign or malignant neoplasm (Table

TABLE 5–3   Classification of Minor Salivary Gland Tumors

Benign
  Mixed tumor
  Oncocytoma
Malignant
  Adenoid cystic carcinoma
  Tumors of duct origin
  Mucoepidermoid carcinoma
  Solid duct carcinoma
  Variants of duct carcinoma
    Mucus adenocarcinoma
    Papillary-cystic carcinoma
    Clear cell
adenocarcinoma
    Papillary adenocarcinoma
    Spindle cell carcinoma
    Unclassified
  Other malignant tumors
    Malignant mixed tumor
    Oat cell carcinoma
    Colonic type carcinoma

Spiro RH, Koss LG, Hajdu SE, Strong EW: Tumors of minor salivary origin: a clinicopathologic study of 492 cases. Cancer 31:117, 1973.

TABLE 5–4   W.H.O. Classification of Salivary Gland Tumors

Epithelial tumors
  Adenomas
    Pleomorphic adenoma (mixed tumor)
  Monomorphic adenomas
    Adenolymphoma
    Oxyphilic adenoma
    Other types
  Mucoepidermoid tumor
  Acinic cell tumor
  Carcinomas
    Adenoid cystic
    Adenocarcinoma
    Epidermoid carcinoma
    Undifferentiated
    Carcinoma in pleomorphic adenoma (malignant
      mixed tumor)
Nonepithelial tumors
Unclassified tumors
Allied conditions
  Benign lymphoepithelial lesion
  Sialosis
  Oncocytosis

Thackray AC, Sobin LH: Histological Typing of Salivary Gland Tumors. Geneva, W.H.O., 1972.

5–1). Malignant degeneration of normal differentiated cells does not occur.

There are a number of different classifications of salivary gland neoplasms. Table 5–2 presents a practical working classification for the clinician. Other classifications are presented in Tables 5–3, 5–4, and 5–5. The term tumor should be avoided in the naming of a neoplasm. Tumor denotes merely a swelling with no connotation of biologic behavior. Rather, their names should clearly spell out whether they are benign or malignant. It is true that in some carcinomas, such as the low- and the intermediate-grade mucoepidermoid carcinomas and all the acinous cell carcinomas, the degree of malignancy cannot be predicted on light microscopic examination, but this does not negate the fact that they are indeed carcinomas.

PLEOMORPHIC ADENOMA

This neoplasm was originally designated the benign mixed tumor in 1866,[10] and its classic microscopic description was given in 1874.[11] A name change to pleomorphic adenoma was first suggested in 1948,[12] and

TABLE 5–5   Soft Tissue Tumors of the Major Salivary Glands and Paraglandular Tissues

Vascular
  Primary hemangioma of the parotid gland
  Lymphangioma
  Arteriovenous fistula (aneurysms)
  Angiosarcoma
Lymphoreticular
  Lymphoma (primary and secondary)
  Atypical lymphoreticular hyperplasia (pseudo-
    lymphoma)
  Histiocytosis
  Lymphoepithelial lesion (with or without Sjögren's
    syndrome)
  Benign reactive hyperplasia
Neurogenous
  Neurofibroma
  Neurofibrosarcoma
  Neurilemmoma
  Traumatic neuroma
  Neuroepithelial tumor (sarcoma)
  Granular cell tumor
  Meningioma
Skeletal muscle
  Rhabdomyosarcoma
  Rhabdomyoma
  Infantile rhabdomyoma
  Masseteric hypertrophy
Smooth muscle
  Leiomyoma
  Leiomyosarcoma
Fibroblastic and histiocytic
  Fibrous scar or keloid
  Fibrosarcoma
  Fibromatosis
  Histiocytoma and variants

considerable controversy has followed. The decision rests on the origin of the myoepithelial cell. The cellular component of a pleomorphic adenoma consists of epidermoid cells and myoepithelial cells. If the two cells have independent origins, the proper name is mixed tumor. If the two cells have a common origin, the proper name is pleomorphic adenoma. Recent evidence favors the latter. Ultrastructural studies suggest that both cells originate from the intercalated duct reserve cell.[8,13] It would also appear that the myoepithelial cell produces the stromal component of the tumor.[13,14] There appears to be a single cell continuum of cytologic featues from the epithelial cell to the mesenchymal cell,[15] and recent histochemical studies further support a unicellular origin. Immunohistochemical studies with antihuman saliva antiserum suggest that the tumor is of epithelial origin from the distal gland cells (intercalated duct reserve cell).[16] Another study showed that the glycoconjugates were the same in the epithelial and the connective tissue components.[17] The final judgment is not in, however, and benign mixed tumor remains in common usage.

Regardless of the name, this neoplasm is the most common of all salivary gland tumors and alone accounts for 65 per cent of parotid, 50 per cent of submandibular, and 30 per cent of minor salivary gland tumors. The latter figure is 93 per cent of all benign tumors of minor salivary gland origin. Ninety per cent of all pleomorphic adenomas occur in the major salivary glands,[18] with 84 per cent occurring in the parotid alone. Ninety per cent of those in the parotid occur in the superficial lobe. Five to 6 per cent arise in the oral cavity, with the palate being the most common site, followed by the tongue. The incidence in the submandibular gland is higher in Africa[20] and in Malaya.[21]

In the major salivary glands, the tumor most commonly appears in the fifth decade, whereas in the minor glands, it appears a decade later. It is slightly more common in women. The average duration before the patient is seen is 6 years. The usual clinical presentation is that of a slow-growing, round, smooth, firm, asymptomatic, mobile mass. The tumor may become lobulated if left untreated. True multicentricity is rare, occurring in 0.5 per cent of all pleomorphic adenomas.[22] A small percentage undergo malignant change if left untreated. This rate has varied from 3[23] to 15 per cent.[24] Signs of malignant change include sudden accelerated growth, facial paralysis, developing irregular margins, fixation to surrounding tissues, or skin ulceration.

Gross examination of a specimen generally reveals a 2- to 5-cm, ovoid, smooth or lobulated, encapsulated mass. The capsule is of varying thickness. Apparent satillitosis is really an outgrowth of the main mass, which can be demonstrated on serial sections.[25] Compression of surrounding tissues is expected and should not be misinterpreted as a sign of malignancy. The cut surface is moist and gray-white, and may have areas of cartilage. Those with a myxoid stroma may have a slimy consistency. Cystic spaces may be present (Figure 5–1).

Microscopically, pleomorphic adenomas are morphologically complex and diverse. There is an epithelial component and a stromal component, and both can be remarkably pleomorphic. The epithelial component consists largely of epithelial and myoepithelial cells, which are classically arranged in a tubular pattern with an inner row of epithelial cells and an outer row of myoepithelial cells. However, the epidermoid cells may be keratinized, and the two cell types may occur in a wide variety of other patterns. The stroma is also pleomorphic and consists of varying admix-

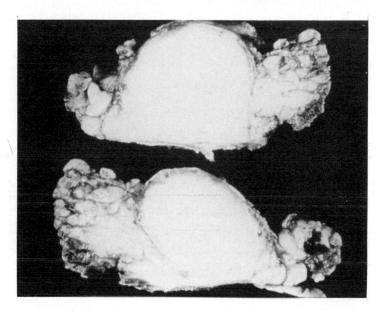

Figure 5–1. Cut surface of pleomorphic adenoma.

tures of mucoid, myxomatous, fibrous, and chondroid areas. Ossification is rare. Tyrosine crystals may be found in the nonepithelial areas and appear to be unique to pleomorphic adenomas.[26] Thirty-six per cent have an equal distribution of myxoid and cellular components (Figure 5–2), whereas 22 per cent are predominantly cellular, and 12 per cent are extremely cellular[27] (Figure 5–3).

Histochemical studies show that the epithelial cells contain PAS-positive mucinous substances, and the stroma contains acid mucopolysaccharides.[28] Chemical analysis of the acid mucopolysaccharides reveals them to be composed of hyaluronic acid and chondrotin sulfate B and C.[29]

The treatment of the pleomorphic adenoma wherever it occurs is complete excision with a cuff of normal tissue around it. Adherence to this policy produces a recurrence rate of less than 5 per cent. For the parotid gland, this requires a minimum of a superficial parotidectomy with preservation of the facial nerve.[30] Others favor routine total parotidectomy with preservation of the facial nerve.[31] A recent report recommending enucleation followed by postoperative irradiation is mentioned only to be condemned.[32] Subjecting a patient to the risks and complications of two modalities of treatment when one carefully executed modality will suffice seems irrational.

The recurrent pleomorphic adenoma deserves special mention. In the past, when enucleation was performed, recurrence rates as high as 50 per

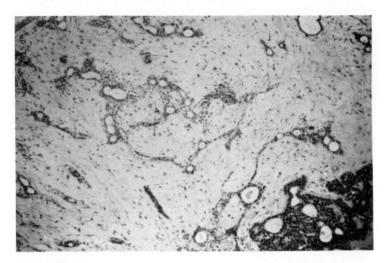

Figure 5–2. Photomicrograph of typical pleomorphic adenoma.

cent were reported, with delays as long as 30 years. Some of these patients are still being seen. Recurrences in the parotid are especially distressing and are usually manifest by multiple nodules in the residual parotid tissue, in the scar, and in the skin. Repeat excision is the treatment of choice and can be a demanding operative procedure. Care must be taken at every step as the nerve may be damaged at the time of flap elevation or any time thereafter, because the previous procedure and subsequent scarring may

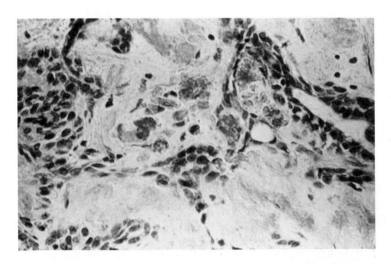

Figure 5–3. Photomicrograph of rather cellular pleomorphic adenoma.

have displaced the nerve from its normal location. The nerve stimulator and the operating microscope can be invaluable in identifying nerve in the midst of scar and recurrent tumor. The surgeon should be prepared to dissect the nerve in either an antegrade or retrograde manner (see Chap. 1). On rare occasions, en bloc removal of the recurrent tumor and the involved portion of the facial nerve may offer the only feasible chance for cure.[33,34] The branch of the facial nerve resected should be immediately repaired. If the situation would require resection of the main trunk of the facial nerve, if the tumor burden is not great, and if the patient is not young, consideration should be given to employing radiation therapy. There is some evidence that radiation often halts the growth of pleomorphic adenomas.[35] If radiation fails, the main trunk can still be resected, particularly since it has been shown that radiation does not interfere with nerve regeneration.[36] It should also be borne in mind that the rate of recurrence accelerates after the first recurrence.[37–39]

WARTHIN'S TUMOR

This entity was first described in 1910[40] in Europe and in 1929[41] in the United States. The designation of adenolymphoma has been adopted by the WHO[27] and the AFIP,[42] but common usage pays homage to Warthin, who reported the first two cases in American literature. In addition, the term adenolymphoma carries a malignant connotation that does not exist with this entity.

The tumor is thought to arise from heterotopic salivary tissue entrapped within a lymph node during embryogenesis, and there is a considerable body of evidence to support this theory.[43–45] Despite a few unquestioned exceptions in the lip and the palate, Warthin's tumor should be viewed as nearly exclusively a parotid or paraparotid disease.[46,47] Most cited exceptions are doubtful.[48]

Eighty-two per cent occur between the ages of 41 and 70 years, with a reported range from 2.5 to 92 years. There is a 5:1 male predominance, and it is rare in blacks and Orientals. It is bilateral in 10 per cent of cases.[19] It accounts for 6 to 10 per cent of parotid tumors and is the second most common benign tumor in the parotid.

The clinical presentation is usually that of a well-defined, soft-to-firm mass in the parotid (Figure 5–4). It is usually 3 to 4 cm in diameter and asymptomatic. However, 18 per cent of patients in one series complained of pain,[49] and there has been one report of facial paralysis.[50] The average duration of the mass on presentation is 3 years. The overwhelming majority of patients are white males, but others are occasionally afflicted, and I have seen bilateral Warthin's tumors in a black female. This tumor scans "hot" with technetium.

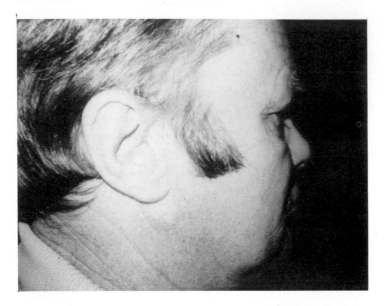

Figure 5–4. Warthin's tumor in tail of right parotid below ear.

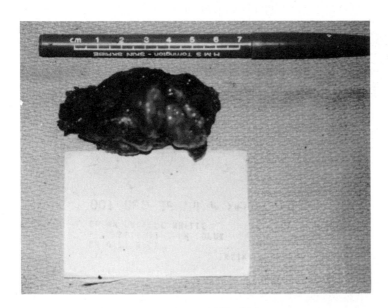

Figure 5–5. Cut surface of Warthin's tumor.

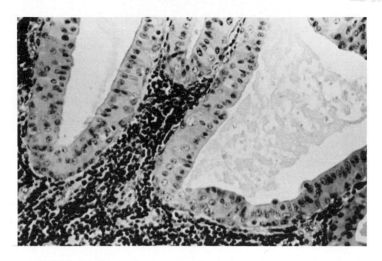

Figure 5–6. Photomicrograph of typical Warthin's tumor.

On gross inspection, the tumor is usually encapsulated, round or oval, cystic, and compressible. Upon sectioning, the tumor is found to contain a mucoid, brown-tinged fluid. The cut surface has multiple irregular cystic spaces with papillary projections (Figure 5–5).

Microscopic examination reveals a double layer of epithelium within a lymphoid stroma containing sinuses and lymphoid follicles. The inner row of epithelial cells has nuclei that are vesicular, whereas those of the outer layer are pyknotic and located toward the luminal surface. The epithelial cells contain abundant mitochondria. Goblet cells may be seen as well as occasional areas of squamous metaplasia (Figure 5–6).

The treatment of Warthin's tumor is excision, usually meaning a superficial parotidectomy. Recurrence rates are essentially unavailable. In one series[24] with reasonable follow-up, 6 of 49 recurred. Recurrences may represent incomplete removal, tumor spillage, or multicentricity, which has been repeatedly reported.

Involvement of Warthin's tumor by lymphoma has been reported and has been shown to be composed of B cells.[51] Epithelial malignancy has been reported in Warthin's tumors in 6 cases. Two cases occurred in patients who had received irradiation to the area for benign conditions 8 and 13 years before.[52,53] All six cases have been recently reviewed.[54]

ONCOCYTOMA

Oncocytes are mutant epithelial cells derived from acini or intralobular ducts. They were originally believed to be the result of a degenerative

TABLE 5–6   Parotid Gland Tumors: Histologic Diagnosis in Reported Cases

Classification	Foote & Frazell (776 cases)	Bardwill (153 cases)	Eneroth (802 cases)	Lambert (83 cases)
	No. (%)	No. (%)	No. (%)	No. (%)
Mixed tumors				
Benign	447(58)	36(34)	569(70.9)	44(53)
Malignant	46(6)	34(22)		1(1)
Warthin's tumor	50(6.5)	5(3)	41(5.1)	16(19)
Mucoepidermoid carcinoma				
Low-grade	45(6)	32(21)	34(4.2)	5(6)
High-grade	45(6)			
Adenoid cystic carcinoma	15(2)	13(8)	19(2.4)	2(2)
Acinous cell carcinoma	21(3)	8(5)	36(4.5)	3(5)
Adenocarcinoma (miscellaneous)	32(4)	16(11)	17(2.1)	
Oncocytic cell tumor	1(0.1)	1(1)	4(0.5)	1(1)
Squamous cell carcinoma	26(3)	8(5)	1(0.1)	1(1)
Miscellaneous				
Benign	3(0.4)			
Malignant	0		15(1.8)	5(6)
Unclassified				
Benign	4(0.6)			
Malignant	30(4)			2(2)

Foote FW Jr, Frazell EL: Tumors of the major salivary glands. Cancer 6:1065, 1953.
Bardwill JM: Tumors of the parotid gland. Am J Surg 114:498, 1969.
Eneroth CM: Histological and clinical aspects of parotid tumors. Acta 'Otolaryngol Suppl 191:1, 1964.
Lambert JA: Parotid gland tumors. Milit Med 136:484, 1971.

process, but recent electron microscopic studies refute this.[55,56] The cells are packed with mitochondria, with an increased but abnormal metabolism producing only small amounts of ATP. Thus oncocytes appear to be a consequence of an acquired disturbance of the mitochondrial enzyme organization. Regardless of the exact underlying cause, oncocytes are normal findings in aging salivary tissue, especially the parotid. Oncocytes are rarely seen before the age of 50 years, but are seen nearly 100% of the time in patients over age 70. Other intracellular organelles may give staining appearances similar to that of the oncocyte, and so the precise documentation of mitochondria must be done by histochemical or electron microscopic means. Further, the precise criteria for the separation of neoplastic and hyperplastic lesions has not been settled.[57] Most oncocytic lesions are probably hyperplasia, not neoplasia.[58]

The oncocytoma was first described in 1875[59] and is believed to account for less than 1 per cent of all salivary gland tumors.[60] It usually occurs in the parotid and is quite unusual elsewhere. In reported series,

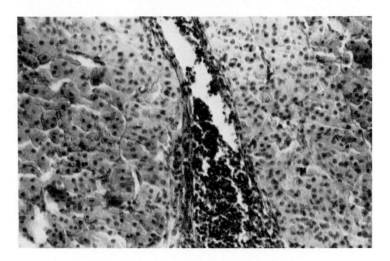

Figure 5–7. Photomicrograph of oncocytoma.

bilaterality and multicentricity have been conspicuous. In concert with the appearance of oncocytes, most tumors occur in the sixth decade. There is a 2:1 female to male ratio. This is one of 2 salivary gland tumors that scans "hot" with technetium. The other is Warthin's tumor.

On gross examination the tumor is encapsulated, lobular, and no greater than 5 cm in diameter. On cut section, it may be solid or papillary. On microscopic examination, the tumor consists of large cells with an eosinophilic-staining granular cytoplasm (Figure 5–7). It is currently impossible to differentiate the benign from the malignant oncocytoma on microscopic examination, but the malignant ones are usually solid.

The treatment is complete excision. Recurrences are uncommon and should be viewed with suspicion, as they may herald a malignant biologic course. Recurrences should be treated quickly and aggressively.

MONOMORPHIC ADENOMAS

The WHO and AFIP classify Warthin's tumor and the oncocytoma as monomorphic adenomas, but most of the literature limits discussion to the lesions that follow—the basal cell adenoma, the membranous adenoma, the salivary duct adenoma, the sebaceous adenoma, the clear cell adenoma, hybrid basal cell adenoma, and the myoepithelioma. Some current articles are more restrictive.[61] The characteristics of monomorphic adenomas are a monomorphic cellular composition, probable origin from the intercalated duct reserve cell, common multicentricity in the major salivary glands, common occurrence in the minor salivary glands, and a benign biologic course. In many monomorphic adenomas there are histologic features that recall stages in the embryology of dermal adnexae, as well as salivary glands. The closest analogous skin tumor is the dermal eccrine cylindroma.[62]

BASAL CELL ADENOMA

This entity was first described in 1967.[63] Through the end of 1981 there had been < 200 cases in the world's literature. The average age is 60, and there is an equal sex distribution. It usually appears as a firm, non-tender, slow-growing mass. There is a distinct predilection for the parotid and for the minor glands in the upper lip, with 80 per cent of minor salivary gland tumors occurring in the upper lip.[64]

On gross examination, a basal cell adenoma is usually round, solid, encapsulated, and less than 3 cm in diameter. On cut section it is grayish-white or grayish-red in color. Microscopic examination reveals isomorphic cells with basophilic staining nuclei and cytoplasm. The cells are arranged in irregular masses or in a trabecular, tubular, or canalicular pattern. The latter may show areas enclosing small blood vessels, a finding that is considered pathognomonic.[65] Some consider the lesion to be the benign

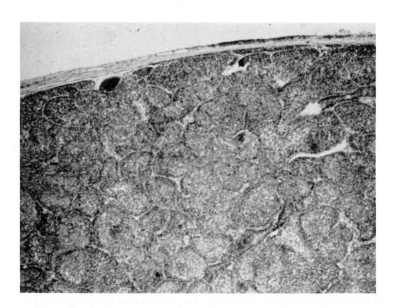

Figure 5–8. Photomicrograph of basal cell adenoma.

variant of the adenoid cystic carcinoma or a "non-pleomorphic" form of the pleomorphic adenoma.[65]

The treatment is excision and recurrences are unexpected.

HYBRID BASAL CELL ADENOMA

This term is used to describe a rare form of basal cell adenoma with histologic features that suggest an evolution toward pleomorphic adenoma or adenoid cystic carcinoma (q.v.). Evolution toward pleomorphic adenoma is more common, but both are so uncommon that predictions about biologic behavior cannot be made. Care must be taken so that this lesion is not misinterpreted as an adenoid cystic carcinoma with its attendant therapeutic implications.

MYOEPITHELIOMA

The myoepithelioma, a rare tumor, is probably a monomorphic varient of the pleomorphic adenoma. The diagnosis is difficult to make and requires electron microscopic demonstration of myoepithelium. There is no sex predilection, and it is clinically indistinguishable from the pleomorphic adenoma.

SEBACEOUS CELL LESIONS

Ectopic sebaceous glands are common within the parotid gland and occur in 33 per cent of adults. They are less common in the other salivary glands. The exact origin of these sebaceous elements is unknown. In addition, sebaceous glands also are commonly found in recognizable salivary gland tumors, especially pleomorphic adenomas, mucoepidermoid carcinomas, and Warthin's tumors.

True neoplasms are unusual and, in decreasing frequency, are the sebaceous lymphadenoma, the sebaceous carcinoma, and the sebaceous adenoma. The sebaceous lymphadenoma is rare and was first described in 1960.[66] The histologic picture is that of sebaceous glands in a lymphoid stroma. The stroma appears identical with that of Warthin's tumor, and the sebaceous lymphadenoma may have a similar origin in parotid nodes. Sebaceous adenomas are extremely rare; a single case was reported in 1954[67] and another in 1959.[68] Both were smooth, round, encapsulated lesions. Excision is curative.

SIALADENOMA PAPILLIFERUM

This lesion was first described in 1969,[69] and there have been 9 reported cases through 1981.[70–72] Like the monomorphic adenomas, this lesion also underscores the similarity between some salivary gland tumors and epidermal appendage tumors. Reported lesions have shown a predilection for the parotid gland and the palate. In the parotid, this lesion appears as a painless, circumscribed mass, whereas on the palate, it has been papillary and exophytic. Microscopic examination reveals papillary folds of epithelium with tortuous, dilated ducts. The epithelial cells that line the papillae may be oxyphilic, mucous, or squamous. All reports have mentioned the similarity of this lesion to syringoadenoma papilliferum. The treatment is excision, and all reported cases have had a benign course.

HEMANGIOMA

The hemangioma accounts for 50 per cent of all parotid tumors in children. It is uncommon in the other salivary glands and in adults. It is of historical interest that the first English language review of the topic was in 1930.[73] The exact nature of these lesions has not been established, but the capillary hemangiomas are probably neoplasms or vascular malformations, whereas the cavernous hemangiomas are best regarded as reactions to trauma or as vascular malformations.[74] The capillary hemangiomas are far more common. There is a modest female predominance. Sixty-one per cent are present at birth, and 86 per cent appear within the first month.[75] They invariably appear as a discrete mass of variable consistency and growth rate. A period of rapid growth, during which the mass may be quite hard, is common at 4 to 6 months of age. The mass is generally painless, transilluminates poorly, and does not have a bruit. There may be an associated cutaneous hemangioma, which lends strong circumstantial evidence for the diagnosis. Fifty per cent show phleboliths on roentgenologic examination.[76]

Gross examination of an excised specimen of a capillary hemangioma reveals a spongy, purple, lobular mass, which infiltrates the gland. Microscopic examination shows endothelial proliferation with vascular differentiation, which is the hallmark of this disease. There are solid masses of cells and multiple anastomosing capillaries surrounding the acini and ducts. Microscopic examination of the cavernous hemangioma reveals dilated blood vessels and sinusoids lined by endothelium. It is unencapsulated and infiltrating (Figure 5–9).

Capillary hemangiomas, which far outnumber the cavernous, have a greater than 90 per cent incidence of spontaneous involution within the first

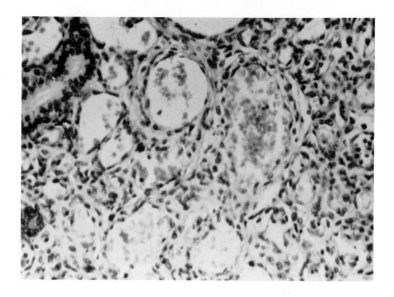

Figure 5–9. Photomicrograph of hemangioma of parotid.

five years of life. If a cutaneous hemangioma is present, they will involute simultaneously, and this is heralded by a central graying of the mass. For this reason, in the absence of a complication, treatment is unnecessary and ill-advised. If complications such as ulceration, hemorrhage, or infection occur, a trial of high dose steroids should be used first. If that fails, and the complications continue without signs of spontaneous involution, excision should be performed. This is best performed after the period of rapid growth if possible, and special precautions should be taken. The facial nerve lies considerably more superficial in the child than in the adult and is easily damaged. In one case the facial nerve was transected during the skin incision. In one series, the mortality was 4.3 per cent and the incidence of facial paralysis was 23 per cent.[77] In another, the recurrance rate was 30 per cent.[78] Radiation therapy is contraindicated. Cavernous hemangiomas do not involute, but the only indications for treatment are the development of a complication or an unacceptable cosmetic deformity. If treatment is deemed necessary, it is probably best delayed until the mastoid tip is well developed and the facial nerve is in a more normal position.

LYMPHANGIOMA

Lymphangiomas (cystic hygromas) were first recognized as being of lymphatic origin in 1828.[79] Their exact method of development is unknown, but they are malformations not true neoplasms. Although greater than 50 per cent of all lymphangiomas occur in the neck, exclusive salivary gland involvement is exceedingly rare. Fifty per cent are present at birth, and 80 to 90 per cent are manifest by the second year of life. They are painless, transilluminate, and usually slowly enlarging. Unlike hemangiomas, less than 15 per cent of lymphangiomas regress substantially. They contain an active lymphaticovenous circulation as demonstrated by xenon-133 that decreases as size increases.[80] There is an equal sex distribution.

Gross examination reveals a spongy, cystic, multiloculated lesion containing fluid that is either clear, cloudy, or yellow-tinged. Microscopic examination demonstrates endothelial lined spaces with a connective tissue stroma.

Treatment is necessary only if vital structures are compromised or if there is an unacceptable cosmetic deformity. Clinically, lymphangiomas occur in one of two forms—a small to medium-sized, unilocular, well circumscribed mass or a diffuse mass with ill-defined margins. The former is rare, but easily excised. The latter can be very difficult to excise completely. When treatment is necessary, as complete an excision as is possible without sacrifice of any vital structures is prudent. Re-excision may be necessary, using the same principles. Radiation, sclerosing agents, and other measures should not be used.

LIPOMA

Lipomas are uncommon in the head and neck and account for 0.6 to 4.4 per cent of all parotid tumors.[81] They are less frequent in the submandibular gland. They most commonly occur in the fifth to sixth decades and are rare in children. There is a 10:1 male to female ratio. Lipomas of the salivary glands, like lipomas that occur elsewhere, are soft, mobile, painless, slow-growing masses.

Gross examination reveals them to be smooth, well-demarcated, and yellow. They may be multilobulated. Microscopic examination shows them to be composed of mature fat cells with an enveloping capsule. Lipomas must be differentiated from diffuse lipomatosis of the parotid.

The treatment is excision. Recurrences are rare and malignant transformation does not occur.

MYXOMA

The true myxoma is an uncommon neoplasm that is rare in the parotid and has not been reported in the other salivary glands. It is a benign

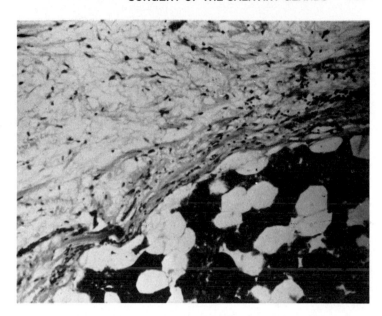

Figure 5–10. Photomicrograph of myxoma of parotid.

mesenchymal tumor that is slow-growing, but infiltrative. It is usually asymptomatic early, but may compress vital structures over time.

Gross examination reveals it to be slimy, mucoid, pallid, and poorly circumscribed. Microscopic examination shows spindle-shaped cells in a myxoid stroma that contains mucopolysaccharide. Within these are delicate reticular fibers.[82] The tumor differs from umbilical cord tissue only in that it may manifest some areas of secondary fibrosis (Figure 5–10).

The treatment is early wide excision. Although slow-growing, the tumor is infiltrative and apt to recur if not widely excised.[83] Radiation is ineffective.

GRANULAR CELL TUMOR

This common tumor of the head and neck is extremely rare in salivary glands.[84] This tumor was originally thought to be of myogenic origin, but recent evidence strongly supports a neurogenic origin.[85] Ten per cent are multiple, either synchronous or metachronous. Grossly, the lesion is circumscribed, but not encapsulated. Microscopic examination reveals polymorphic cells with pale-staining, acidophilic, and granular cytoplasm. In the more common, submucosal locations, it is often covered by pseudoepitheliomatous hyperplasia. The treatment is wide excision since it is not encapsulated. They are also benign and radiation is ineffective.

SCHWANNOMA

Schwannoma is currently the preferred term for a benign nerve sheath tumor also termed the neurilemoma, the neurolemmoma and other less accurate names.[86] These are not true salivary gland tumors, but on rare occasion do involve the facial nerve within the parotid. The first reported case was in 1930,[87] and there have been less than 30 cases reported since. The tumors are slow-growing with an equal sex distribution. Paresthesias are common, as is tenderness. Fifty per cent of these patients have facial weakness when first seen.

Gross examination reveals a glistening, white, encapsulated mass. Microscopic examination reveals a tumor composed of Schwann cells with frequent degenerative changes, such as cyst formation and hemorrhagic necrosis. The Schwann cells occur in two distinctive patterns. In the Antoni A pattern the nuclei palisade around a central area of cytoplasm (the Verocay body). In the Antoni B type the cells are arranged in no particular pattern. Both areas usually occur in the same tumor.

The tumor tends to push axons aside rather than incorporate them. Malignant degeneration does not occur. For these reasons, during excision an attempt should be made to preserve the facial nerve as much as possible. Radiation is ineffective.

NEUROFIBROMA

This tumor also arises from the Schwann cell, but behaves much differently. The tumor is unencapsulated, and may be solitary or part of neurofibromatosis. The former is much more common. Axons are incorporated into the tumor, and approximately 8 per cent undergo malignant change. Fortunately neurofibromas tend to be centrifugally located, and involvement of the facial nerve within the parotid is exceedingly rare. Preservation of the facial nerve is impossible during excision, since the nerve is incorporated into the tumor.

TERATOMA

Teratomas are neoplasms composed of multiple tissues foreign to the part of the body in which they arise. In the head and neck they are pathologic curiosities, and are exceedingly rare in the parotid[88] and unreported in the other salivary glands. The treatment is excision.

BENIGN NEOPLASMS IN CHILDREN

Salivary epithelial neoplasms in children are rare. They constitute less than 5 per cent of all salivary tumors.[89,90] Fifty per cent are benign. At least 85% of benign neoplasms are pleomorphic adenomas.[91] However, pleomorphic adenomas in children account for only 1.4% of all pleomorphic adenomas.[92] The second most common benign neoplasm is Warthin's tumor, which accounts for 2 to 3%. Of 132 Warthin's tumors in one series,[93] only 4 occurred in children. The vast majority of benign neoplasms occur in the parotid gland, and the peak age incidence is 10 years. Parotidectomy with preservation of the facial nerve is the preferred treatment. Some have expressed an increased recurrence rate for the pleomorphic adenoma, but this may merely reflect a conservative operative procedure.

SUBMANDIBULAR, SUBLINGUAL, AND MINOR SALIVARY GLAND TUMORS

The same benign tumors that occur in the parotid gland also occur in the other salivary glands. The statistics, however, are dominated by the pleomorphic adenoma and the basal cell adenoma. The others are exceed-

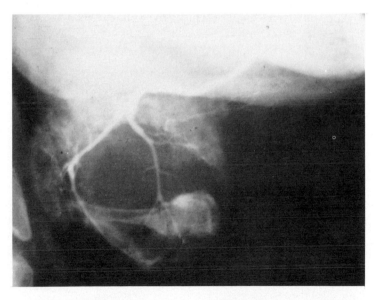

Figure 5–11. Sialogram showing ducts draping around pleomorphic adenoma of submandibular gland.

ingly rare. The biologic behavior remains benign and complete excision is curative.

The submandibular gland is the site of 10 per cent of all salivary gland neoplasms. Forty per cent of these are pleomorphic adenomas (Figure 5–11). There is a 2:1 female to male predominance. Since the tumors are often inconspicuous, asymptomatic, and slow-growing, the duration of the mass prior to treatment often exceeds 5 years. Complete excision of the submandibular gland is usually curative. The recurrence rate is 5 to 6 per cent, and these invariably follow inadequate excision.[89]

The sublingual gland is the site of 0.5 to 4.5 per cent of all salivary gland tumors. To date there have been less than 50 cases of benign tumors reported, underscoring the fact that at least 80 per cent are malignant. The benign tumors are virtually exclusively pleomorphic adenomas, which occur as an asymptomatic mass under the anterior tongue. Complete excision of this gland is curative, and there have been no recurrences.

Minor salivary glands are distributed widely in the upper respiratory tract. The most common location for minor salivary gland tumors is the oral cavity. In the oral cavity, the most common location is the palate for benign tumors (Figure 5–12), followed by the upper lip and the buccal mucosa.[90] In the palate itself, the most common location is the posterior one-third of the hard palate and the soft palate. This corresponds to the location of the minor salivary glands, which are uncommon anterior to a line connecting the first molars.[91] The lesion, in all locations, appears as an asymptomatic, submucosal swelling usually present for months. Except for those on the palate, they are usually mobile. Pleomorphic adenomas

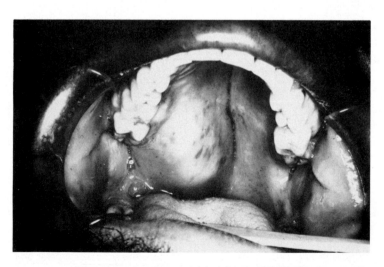

Figure 5–12. Pleomorphic adenoma of palate.

account for 56 per cent of all minor salivary gland intraoral tumors.[92] Second in frequency is the basal cell adenoma. Mangement is by wide excision.[93] Although intraoral benign tumors are usually not encapsulated, recurrences with adequate excision occur in approximately 10 per cent.[94]

Minor salivary gland neoplasms account for 4 to 8 per cent of all neoplasms of the nose and paranasal sinuses. Most are malignant, with the pleomorphic adenoma being third in frequency, behind the adenoid cystic carcinoma and the adenocarcinoma. All other benign neoplasms are quite unusual. The pleomorphic adenoma is usually intranasal rather than intrasinus, and most often arises from the nasal septum. Twenty per cent arise from the lateral nasal wall. The presenting symptom is usually nasal airway obstruction; epistaxis is uncommon. There is an equal sex distribution. The treatment is complete excision, and recurrences are uncommon.

The larynx and trachea are uncommon sites for benign salivary gland neoplasms. Essentially all reported cases are pleomorphic adenomas. When they occur in the supraglottis they usually cause a voice change. When they occur in the subglottis or trachea, they usually cause airway obstruction. Pleomorphic adenomas are more common in the trachea than in the larynx, with more than 25 cases reported in the former.[95]

On rare occasions benign tumors occur in aberrant salivary gland tissue. Aberrant salivary gland tissue has been reported in tonsils in 1 per cent of cases, is common in the pituitary, and has been reported in the mandible, lower neck, middle ear, along the thyroglossal duct, and in the sternoclavicular joint. Pleomorphic adenomas are quite rare in the mandible, and there has been one reported case in the middle ear.[96]

REFERENCES

1. Eneroth CM: Histological and clinical aspects of parotid tumors. Acta Otolaryngol (Suppl) 191:1, 1964.
2. Batsakis JG: Tumors of the Head and Neck. Baltimore, Williams & Wilkins, 1979, p. 1.
3. Thackray AC: Salivary gland tumors. Proc R Soc Med 61:1089, 1968.
4. Eneroth CM: Incidence and prognosis of salivary gland tumors at different sites. A study of parotid, submandibular, and palatal tumors in 2632 patients. Acta Orolaryngol 263:174, 1970.
5. Eneroth DM: Salivary gland tumors of the parotid gland, submandibular gland, and the palate region. Cancer 27:1415, 1971.
6. Edington GM, Sheiham A: Salivary gland tumors and tumors of the oral cavity in Western Nigeria. Br J Cancer 20:20, 1966.
7. Eversole LR: Histogenic classification of salivary tumors. Arch Pathol 92:433, 1971.
8. Regezi JA, Batsakis JG: Histogenesis of salivary gland neoplasms. Otolaryngol Clin N Amer 10:297, 1977.
9. Pierce GB: Neoplasms, differentiations and mutations. Am J Pathol 77:103, 1974.
10. Broca P: Traté des Tumeurs. Paris, P. Asselin, 1866.
11. Menissen H: Uber gemischte Geschwulste der Parotis. Dissertation. 1874.
12. Cited in Willis RA: Pathology of Tumors. St. Louis, C. V. Mosby Company, 1953.

13. Hubner, G, Kleinsasser O, Klein JH: Zur Feinstruktur der Speichelgangearcinome. Virchow's Arch 346:1, 1968.
14. Kleinsasser O: Einteilung, morphologie und verhalten der epithelialen speicheldrusen-tumoren. HNO 17:197, 1969.
15. Mills SE, Cooper PH: An ultrastructural study of cartilaginous zones and surrounding epithelium in mixed tumors of salivary glands and skin. Lab Invest 44:6, 1981.
16. Vigliani R, Stramignoni A: Cytologic localization of antigens from human saliva in pleomorphic adenomas of salivary glands. Cancer 48 (2, Suppl):293, 1981.
17. Rovasio RA, Ronseca MM, Gendelman H, Monis B: Histochemistry of glycoconjugates of pleomorphic adenomas of minor salivary glands, with special reference to glycocalyx of tubular areas. Oral Surg 50:58, 1980.
18. Rauch S: Die Speicheldrusen des Menschen. Stuttgart, Georg Thieme, 1959.
19. Rauch S, Seifert G, Gorlin RJ: Diseases of the salivary glands: tumors. In Gorlin RH, Goldman HM (eds): Thoma's Oral Pathology. St. Louis, C. V. Mosby Company, 1970.
20. Davies JNP, Dodge OG, Burkitt DP: Salivary gland tumors in Uganda. Cancer 17:1310, 1964.
21. Marsden ATH: The distinctive features of the tumours of the salivary glands in Malaya. Br J Cancer 5:375, 1951.
22. Batsakis JG: Tumors of the Head and Neck. Baltimore, Williams & Wilkins, 1979, p. 25.
23. Eneroth CM: Classification of parotid tumors. Proc R Soc Med 59:429, 1966.
24. Foote FW Jr, Frazell EL: Tumors of the major salivary glands. Cancer 6:1065, 1953.
25. Eneroth CM: Mixed tumors of major salivary glands: prognostic role of capsular struc-ture. Ann Otol Rhinol Laryngol 74:944, 1965.
26. Thomas K, Hutt MS: Tyrosine crystals in salivary gland tumors. J Clin Pathol 34:1003, 1981.
27. Thackray AC, Sobin LH: Histological Typing of Salivary Gland Tumors. Geneva, WHO, 1972.
28. Grishman E: Histochemical analysis of mucopolysaccharides occurring in mucus-pro-ducing tumors: mixed tumors of the parotid glands, colloid carcinomas of the breast, and myxomas. Cancer 5:700, 1952.
29. Lovell D, Briggs JC, Schorah CJ: Chemical analysis of acid mucopolysaccharides of mixed salivary tumors. Br J Cancer 20:463, 1966.
30. Boles R: Parotid neoplasms: surgical treatment and complications. Otolaryngol Clin N Amer 10:413, 1977.
31. Work WP: The recurrent mixed tumor. Otolaryngol Clin N Amer 10:427, 1977.
32. Armitstead RP, Smiddy FG, Frank HG: Simple enucleation and radiotherapy in the treatment of pleomorphic salivary adenoma of the parotid gland. Br J Surg 66:716, 1979.
33. Work WP, Batsakis JG, Bailey DH: Recurrent benign mixed tumor and the facial nerve. Arch Otolaryngol 102:15, 1976.
34. Conley J, Clairmont AA: Facial nerve in recurrent benign pleomorphic adenoma. Arch Otolaryngol 105:247, 1979.
35. Piorkowski RJ, Guillamandegui OM: Is aggressive surgical treatment indicated for recur-rent benign mixed tumors of the parotid gland. Am J Surg 142:434, 1981.
36. McGuirt WF, McCabe BF: Effect of radiation therapy in facial nerve cable autografts. Laryngoscope 87:415, 1977.
37. Grage TB, Lober PH, Shanon DB: Benign tumors of the major salivary glands. Surgery 50:625, 1961.
38. Winsten J, Ward GE: Mixed tumors of the parotid gland. Surgery 42:1029, 1957.
39. Molnar L, Ronay P, Dobrossy L: Mixed tumours of the parotid gland. Oncology 25:143, 1971.
40. Albrecht H, Arzt L: Beitrage zur frage der gewebsverirrung. I. Papillare cystadenome in lymphdrusen. Frankf Z Path 4:47, 1910.
41. Warthin AS: Papillary cystadenoma lymphomatosum. A rare teratoid of the parotid region. J Cancer Res 13:116, 1929.
42. Thackray AC, Lucas RB: Tumors of the major salivary glands. Atlas of Tumor Pathol-

ogy, Second Series, Fascicle 10, Armed Forces Institute of Pathology, Washington, DC, 1974.
43. Feyrter F: Uber das onkozytom der speicheldrusen. Zentralbl Allg Pathol 104:513, 1963.
44. Thompson AS, Bryant HC: Histogenesis of papillary cystadenoma lymphomatosum (Warthin's tumor) of the parotid gland. Am J Pathol 26:807, 1950.
45. Azzopardi JG, Horr LT: The genesis of adenolymphoma. J Pathol Bacteriol 88:213, 1964.
46. Cohen MA, Batsakis JG: Warthin's tumor revisited. Mich Med 67:1341, 1968.
47. Kleinsasser O, Klein JH, Steinback E, Hubner G: Onkocytare adenomastige hyperplasien, adenolymphome und onkocytome der speicheldritsen. Arch Klin Exper Ohr Nos Kehlkopj 186:317, 1966.
48. Batsakis JG: Tumors of the Head and Neck. Baltimore, Williams & Wilkins, 1979, p. 55.
49. McGurk FM, Main JHP, Orr JA: Adenolymphoma of the parotid gland. Br J Surg 57:321, 1970.
50. Wilkie TF, White RA: Benign parotid tumor with facial nerve paralysis. Plast Reconstr Surg 43:528, 1969.
51. Cossman J, Deegan MJ, Batsakis JG: Warthin tumor: B-lymphocytes within the lymphoid infiltrate. Arch Pathol Lab Med 101:354, 1977.
52. Little JW, Rickles NH: Malignant papillary cystadenoma lymphomatosum: report of a case with a review of the literature. Cancer 18:1851, 1965.
53. De La Pava S, Knutson GH, Mukhtar F, Pickren JW: Squamous cell carcinoma arising in Warthin's tumor of the parotid gland: first case report. Cancer 18:790, 1965.
54. McClatchey KD, Appelblatt NH, Langin JL: Carcinoma in papillary cystadenoma lymphomatosum (Warthin's tumor). Laryngoscope 42:98, 1982.
55. Askew JB Jr, Fechner RE, Bentinck DC, Jenson AB: Epithelial and myoepithelial oncocytes: Ultrastructural study of a salivary gland oncocytoma. Arch Otolaryngol 93:46, 1971.
56. Tandler B: Fine structure of oncocytes in human salivary glands. Virchow's Arch (Pathol Anat) 341:317, 1966.
57. Tandler B, Hutter RVP, Erlandson RA: Ultrastructure of oncocytoma of the parotid gland. Lab Invest 23:567, 1970.
58. Batsakis JG: Tumors of the Head and Neck. Baltimore, Williams & Wilkins, 1979, p. 60.
59. Duplay M: Adenome de la gland sousmaxillaire. Arch Gen Med 1:601, 1875.
60. Sohn D: Oxyphil adenoma (oncocytoma) of parotid with hemorrhage: Presentation as an enlarging neck mass. EENT Mon 53:242, 1974.
61. Batsakis JG, Brannon RB, Sciubba JJ: Monomorphic adenomas of major salivary glands: a histologic study of 96 tumors. Clin Otolaryngol 6:129, 1981.
62. Batsakis JG, Brannon RB: Dermal analogue tumors of major salivary glands. J Laryngol Otol 95:155, 1981.
63. Kleinsasser O, Klein HJ: Basalzelladenome der speicheldrussen. Arch Klein Exp Ohr Nors Kelkop 189:312, 1967.
64. Fantasia JE, Neville BW: Basal cell adenomas of the minor salivary glands. A clinicopathologic study of seventeen new cases and a review of the literature. Oral Surg 50:433, 1980.
65. Bernacki EG, Batsakis JG, Johns ME: Basal cell adenoma. Distinctive tumor of salivary glands. Arch Otolaryngol 99:84, 1974.
66. McGavran MH, Bauer WC, Ackerman LV: Sebaceous lymphadenoma of the parotid salivary gland. Cancer 13:1185, 1960.
67. Foote FW, Frazell EL: Tumors of the major salivary glands. Atlas of Tumor Pathology. Fascicle 11, Washington DC, Armed Forces Institute of Pathology, 1954.
68. Rauch S, Masshoff W: Die Talgdrusenahnlichen sialome. Frank FZ: Path 68:513, 1959.
69. Abrams AM, Finck FM: Sialadenoma papilliferum. A previously unreported salivary gland tumor. Cancer 24:1057, 1969.
70. Freedman PD, Lumerman H: Sialadenoma papilliferum. Oral Surg 45:88, 1978.

71. McCoy JM, Eckert EF Jr: Sialadenoma papilliferum. J Oral Surg 38:691, 1980.
72. Nasu M, Takagi M, Ishikawa G: Sialadenoma papilliferum: report of case. J Oral Surg 39:367, 1981.
73. McFarland JH: Congenital papillary angioma of the parotid: consideration of similar cases in literature. Arch Pathol 9:820, 1930.
74. Batsakis JG: Tumors of the Head and Neck. Baltimore, Williams & Wilkins, 1979, p. 66.
75. Goldman RC, Perzik SL: Infantile hemangioma of the parotid gland. Arch Otolaryngol 90:605, 1969.
76. Herbert G, Oumet-Oliva D, Ladouceur J: Vascular tumors of the salivary glands in children. Am J Roentgenol Rad Ther Nucl Med 123:815, 1975.
77. Wolfe JJ: Congenital hemangioma of the parotid gland. Plast Reconstr Surg 29:692, 1962.
78. Wowro NW, Fredrickson, RW, Tennant R: Hemangioma of the parotid gland in the newborn and infancy. Cancer 8:595, 1955.
79. Redenbacher cited in Ward PH, Harris PF, Douney W: Surgical approach to cystic hygroma of the neck. Arch Otolaryngol 91:508, 1970.
80. Tonlonkian RJ, Rickert RR, Lange RC, Spencer RP: The microvascular circulation of lymphangiomas. A study of Xe^{133} clearance and pathology. Pediatrics 48:36, 1971.
81. Walts AE, Perzik SL: Lipomatous lesions of the parotid area. Arch Otolaryngol 102:230, 1976.
82. Stout AP: Myxoma: the tumor of primative mesenchyme. Ann Surg 127:706, 1948.
83. Canalis RE, Smith GS, Konrad HR: Myxomas of the head and neck. Arch Otolaryngol 102:176, 1976.
84. Nussbaum M, Haselkorn A: Granular-cell myoblastoma in parotid gland. NY State J Med 72:2887, 1972.
85. Fisher ER, Wechsler H: Granular cell myoblastoma—a misnomer. Electron microscopic and histochemical evidence concerning its Schwann cell derivation and nature (granular cell schwannoma). Cancer 15:936, 1962.
86. Batsakis JG: Tumors of the Head and Neck. Baltimore, Williams & Wilkins, 1979, p. 314.
87. Schmidt C: Neurinam des N Facialis. Zurich, Johres versammund der Gesellscheft Schweizep Hals und Ohrenartz, 1930, p. 52.
88. Shadid EA, O'Neal E, Glass RT: Benign teratoid of the parotid. Plast Reconstr Surg 53:363, 1975.
89. Eneroth CM, Hjertman L: Benign tumors of the submandibular gland. Pract Otorhinolaryngol 29:166, 1967.
90. Frable WJ, Elzoy RP: Tumors of minor salivary glands: a report of 73 cases. Cancer 25:932, 1970.
91. Coates HLC, Devine KD, DeSanto LW, Weiland LH: Glandular tumors of the palate. Surg Gynec Obstet 140:589, 1975.
92. Chaudry AP, Vickers RA, Gorlin RJ: Intraoral minor salivary gland tumors: an analysis of 1414 cases. Oral Surg 14:194, 1961.
93. Worthington P: The management of the palatal pleomorphic adenoma. Br J Oral Surg 12:132, 1974.
94. Eneroth CM, Hjertman L, Moberger G: Salivary gland adenomas of the palate. Acta Otolaryngol 73:305, 1972.
95. Ma CK, Fine G, Lewis L, Lee MW: Benign mixed tumor of the trachea. Cancer 44:2260, 1979.
96. Saeed YM, Bassis MC: Mixed tumor of the middle ear: a case report. Arch Otolaryngol 93:433, 1971.

Chapter Six

MALIGNANT NEOPLASMS

GENERAL CONSIDERATIONS

Malignant neoplasms of the salivary glands occur far less commonly than benign neoplasms. Approximately 1 of 6 parotid, 1 of 3 submandibular, 1 of 2 minor salivary gland, and 4 of 5 sublingual gland neoplasms will be malignant.[1] In general terms, disregarding specific histologic types, the prognosis is most favorable for those located on the palate, less favorable in the parotid, and least favorable in the submandibular gland.[2] Their behavior is best described by Ackerman and del Regato, "The usual tumor of salivary gland is a tumor in which the benign variant is less benign than the usual benign tumor and the malignant variant is less malignant than the usual malignant tumor."[3] For this reason, the success of any treatment program is best evaluated after 20 years rather than 5 or 10 years.

The majority of malignant salivary neoplasms occur in the fifth and sixth decades, although 2 per cent occur in children 1 to 10 years of age, and 16 per cent occur in those less than 30 years of age. There is no general sexual predilection. It is usually difficult on clinical grounds alone to determine whether a salivary gland tumor is benign or malignant. Sixty[4] to 85 per cent[5] appear as a mass with no other associated signs or symptoms. In the minor salivary glands, the most common location is the palate, followed by the tongue.[6] Fifty per cent of intraoral salivary neoplasms occur on the palate. The presence or absence of pain does not help in distinguishing the benign from the malignant. In 5 per cent of benign and 6 per cent of malignant salivary neoplasms, pain is associated with the mass.[7] However, if the tumor is malignant, the presence of pain considerably worsens the prognosis. For those malignant tumors with pain the overall 5 year survival is 33 per cent, whereas for those without pain it is 66 per cent.[8] Others have found a similar adverse effect.[9] Facial nerve paralysis on presentation indicates a grave prognosis and occurs in 12 to 14 per cent of parotid carcinomas. In one large series, the 5-year mortality was 100 per cent;[10] in another it was 86 per cent.[11] In the latter series, all the survivors had low-grade mucoepidermoid carcinomas. Distant metastases were once believed to be uncommon, but this is probably not the case. It is now clear that as the length of follow-up increases, so does the incidence of distant metastases. The presence of local control does not

TABLE 6–1 Staging System for Cancers of the Salivary Glands (American Joint Committee on Cancer, 1980)

Primary Tumor
    TX Tumor cannot be assessed
    TO No evidence of primary tumor
    T1 Tumor less than 2.0 cm in diameter without significant local extension (into skin, bone, soft tissues, or lingual or facial nerves)
    T2 Tumor 2.0 to 4.0 cm in diameter without significant local extension
    T3 Tumor 4.0 to 6.0 cm in diameter without significant local extension
    T4a Tumor over 6.0 cm in diameter without significant local extension
    T4b Tumor of any size with significant local extension
Nodal Involvement
    NX Nodes cannot be assessed
    NO No evidence of regional node involvement
    N1 Clinically or histologically positive regional nodes
Distant Metastasis
    MX Not assessed
    MO No known distant metastasis
    M1 Distant metastasis present
Stage Grouping
    Stage I   T1 NO MO
               T2 NO MO
    Stage II T3 NO MO
    Stage III T1 or T2 NO MO
               T4a or T4b NO MO
    Stage IV T3 N1 MO
               T4a or T4b N1 MO
               Any T, any N, M1

necessarily prevent the later occurrence of distant metastases. The lungs are the most common site, followed by the bones.

The overall recurrence rate for salivary carcinomas varies from 27 per cent[9] to 50 per cent.[12] The incidence of salivary neoplasia, especially of the parotid, is increased after exposure to low- and medium-dose irradiation.[13] The latency period averages 25 years, and the incidence of neoplasia increases with time. Women who have a salivary gland cancer have a significantly increased risk of developing breast cancer, with the converse also being true.[14,15] As many as 11 per cent of patients with a salivary gland cancer present with a simultaneous second malignancy.[4]

The clinical staging of salivary gland cancers, as currently recommended by the American Joint Committee on Cancer, is shown in Table 6–1. This classification system is based on a large retrospective study involving 11 United States and Canadian institutions.[16] Figures 6–1 through 6–4 show the cumulative survival percentages using the TNM criteria proposed in this study.

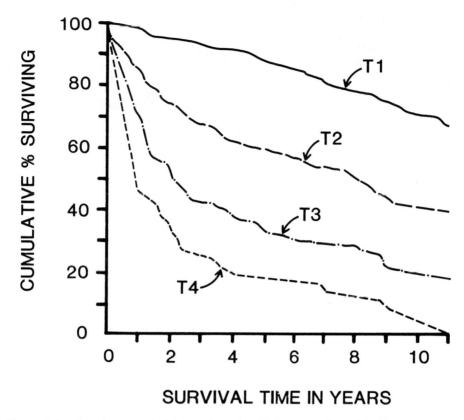

Figure 6–1. Cumulative survival figures for various T sizes regardless of the histologic type of tumor.

The remainder of this chapter will deal with specific neoplasms, with sections on the submandibular, sublingual, and minor salivary glands, and on controversial treatment modalities.

MUCOEPIDERMOID CARCINOMA

The first reported case of mucoepidermoid carcinoma was in 1895.[17] This neoplasm received its current name in 1945,[18] which is based on the two main cellular components noted on microscopic examination—mucous cells and epidermoid cells. The tumor arises from the excretory duct reserve cell. (See section on histogenesis in Benign Neoplasms.)

The mucoepidermoid carcinoma accounts for 3 to 9 per cent of all salivary gland tumors,[19,20] and 7 to 29 per cent of all malignant salivary

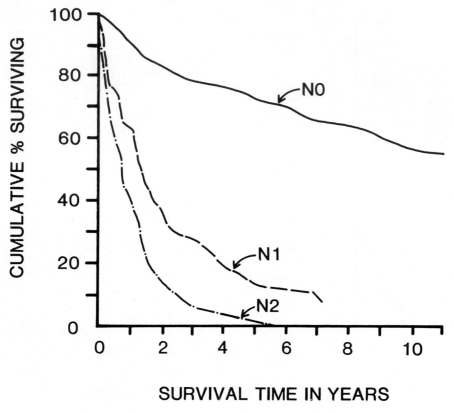

Figure 6–2. Cumulative survival figures for various N sizes regardless of the histologic type of the tumor.

gland tumors.[4,5] It is the most common malignant neoplasm of the parotid gland[21] and accounts for 21 per cent of parotid malignant neoplasms. Sixty to 70 per cent of all mucoepidermoid carcinomas occur in the parotid gland, and this type accounts for 10 per cent of all intraoral minor salivary gland tumors and 26 per cent of all malignant ones. The palate is the second most common location for mucoepidermoid carcinomas.

Although once considered to exist in benign and malignant forms, all mucoepidermoid tumors are currently believed to be carcinomas. They are currently divided into low, intermediate, and high grades based on the microscopic appearance. Low-grade tumors have numerous mucous cells and cystic spaces (Figure 6–5). High-grade tumors resemble squamous cell carcinomas with few mucous cells. Keratinization may occur. Intermediate tumors are intermediate in appearance. Generally biologic behavior parallels microscopic appearance, but this is not always true. Some low-grade

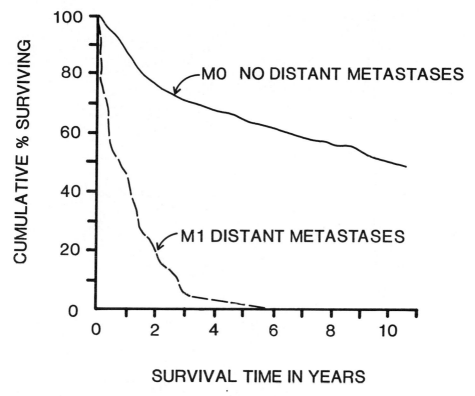

Figure 6–3. Cumulative survival figures for M0 and M1 patients regardless of the histologic type of the tumor.

tumors may behave aggressively and the converse may be true for occasional high-grade carcinomas. From a clinical standpoint, the intermediate classification is not helpful, because most behave like the low-grade tumors. It may be possible to more accurately predict biologic behavior by determining the DNA content. Tumors with a diploid DNA content tend to be noninvasive, whereas those with a triploid DNA content are liable to aggressive behavior.[22,23] Seventy-five per cent of mucoepidermoid carcinomas are low grade.

On gross examination, the low-grade tumors are usually circumscribed, but not encapsulated. High-grade carcinomas tend to have less well-defined margins. The tumors are firm to hard and gray-white to gray-red in color. The cut surface may have cysts, especially in the low-grade neoplasms. Microscopically the tumor is composed of varying percentages of 6 cell types. The maternal cell is the progenitor of the other 5. The intermediate cell may differentiate into either glandular or epidermoid

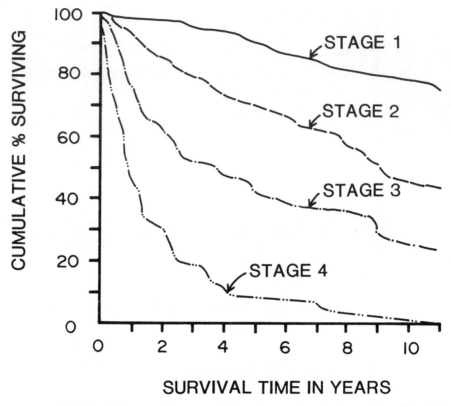

Figure 6–4. Cumulative survival figures for the various stages regardless of the histologic type of the tumor.

forms. The epidermoid cell may closely resemble squamous cell carcinoma with individual cell keratinization, keratin pearls, and intracellular bridges. The clear cell has a distinct outline with hydropic, water-clear cytoplasm. The columnar cell resembles cells found in the major secreting ducts. The sixth cell is the mucous cell.

Most low-grade mucoepidermoid carcinomas appear as a mass indistinguishable from a pleomorphic adenoma. The majority occur in the fourth to sixth decades with a long history, usually months to years. There is a slight female predominance. Up to 8 per cent appear with facial nerve paralysis.[4] Ten per cent or less ever develop metastases. In general, adequate treatment is by wide excision. In the parotid, this usually allows preservation of the facial nerve if it is not involved. The recurrence rate is 15 per cent,[19] and recurrences should be treated aggressively, as the biologic behavior may belie the benign microscopic appearance. The overall 5-year survival is greater than 90 per cent.

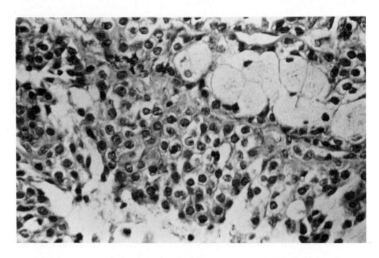

Figure 6–5. Photomicrograph of low-grade mucoepidermoid carcinoma.

The high-grade mucoepidermoid carcinoma usually has a shorter history. The margins are usually less distinct on palpation (Figure 6–6). As many as 25 per cent of patients have preoperative facial paralysis, and 50 per cent have cervical metastases. There is divergence of opinion as to the correct treatment for high-grade mucoepidermoid carcinomas. Some favor a conservative operative approach with preservation of the facial nerve

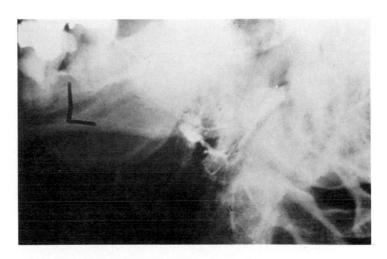

Figure 6–6. Sialogram demonstrating extravasation of contrast material in high grade mucoepidermoid carcinoma.

unless it is involved.[5] Others prefer a radical procedure, such as a radical parotidectomy with sacrifice of the facial nerve, resection of the underlying muscles, and a radical neck dissection as the standard operative procedure.[4] Both schools of thought tend to use postoperative radiation therapy. Published recurrence rates vary from 30 per cent[2,20] to 60 per cent to 75 per cent.[5] There is little difference in the 5-year survivals for the conservative approach (83 per cent) and the more radical approach (78 per cent). Other large series[24] report lower survivals (41 per cent). Much of the difference may relate to different classifications by the pathologist or a different patient population. It seems rational that the operative procedure be designed to remove the entire tumor with a margin of normal tissue around it. It seems unnecessary to sacrifice the facial nerve unless it is involved or to do a radical neck dissection unless palpable adenopathy is present. This is particularly true if postoperative radiation therapy is planned. As with most salivary gland carcinomas, survival figures are worse in the minor glands, with palate lesions yielding a 17 per cent 5-year survival.[25] In one series survival was reported by stage rather than by microscopic appearance, with 5-year survivals of 100 per cent for stage I, 65 per cent for stage II, and 10 per cent for stage III.[9]

ADENOID CYSTIC CARCINOMA

The name adenoid cystic carcinoma was coined in 1953.[26] This tumor was originally designated cylindroma in 1859.[27] The latter term is too nonspecific and should be discarded.[2] It accounts for 4 per cent of all neoplasms of the major salivary glands and 2 to 5 per cent of all parotid tumors. However, it comprises 35 per cent of all malignant minor salivary gland tumors and 40 to 60 per cent of all sublingual gland tumors[4] (Figure 6–7). It is the most common malignant tumor of the submandibular gland.

There is an equal sexual and racial distribution, and the mean age at presentation is 45 years. The majority appear as an asymptomatic mass with a duration of 4 weeks to 20 years.[28] Twenty per cent appear with paresthesias.[4] Thirty per cent have partial or total facial paralysis initially.[29] This high percentage of early facial paralysis graphically demonstrates the propensity to perineural invasion, which is the hallmark of this carcinoma[30] (Figure 6–8).

On gross inspection, the adenoid cystic carcinoma is usually unilobular, 2 to 4 cm in diameter, and circumscribed. The cut surface is moist and grey-pink. Microscopic examination shows the tumor to be unencapsulated, with microscopic extensions that belie the appearance of being circumscribed. The tumor is composed of uniform basaloid cells with scant cytoplasm and regular nuclei. The cells are classically arranged in a

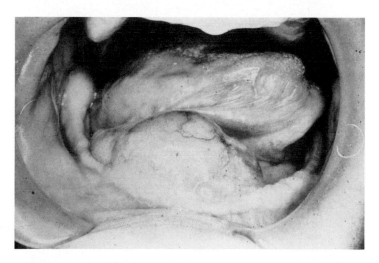

Figure 6–7. Adenoid cystic carcinoma of the sublingual gland in an 83-year-old woman.

cribriform or Swiss cheese pattern (Figure 6–9), but a variety of other patterns occur (Figure 6–10). The cystic spaces are not true cysts, but are extracellular spaces lined by replicated basement membrane. The stroma is also quite variable, but is often myxoid. In the past, some have attempted to relate survival to the histologic appearance, but it is now believed that there is no relationship.[31–34]

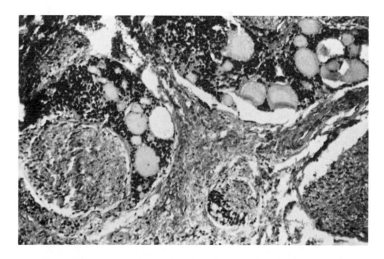

Figure 6–8 Photomicrograph of adenoid cystic carcinoma showing perineural invasion.

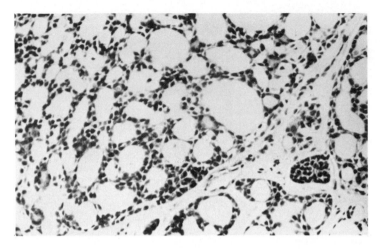

Figure 6–9. Photomicrograph of adenoid cystic carcinoma showing cribriform pattern.

Adenoid cystic carcinomas display a wide diversity of biologic behavior. Some are rapidly fatal; others run an extremely protracted course. This makes an assessment of treatment results difficult, and 5- and 10-year survival figures are of limited value. Fifteen- and 20-year follow-ups are more meaningful because the long-term prognosis is grave. In one study,[4] at 5 years, 3 per cent of the survivors had metastases and local recurrence,

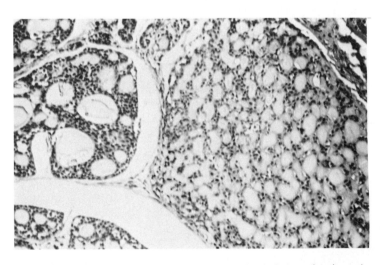

Figure 6–10. Photomicrograph of adenoid cystic carcinoma showing cylindromatous pattern.

TABLE 6–2   Survival of Adenoid Cystic Carcinoma by Site of Origin

Site	10-Year Cure (%)
Parotid	29
Orval cavity	23
Submandibular gland	10
Paranasal sinuses	7

3 per cent had local recurrence only, and 18 per cent had metastases only. At 10 years, 25 per cent of the survivors had metastases and local recurrence, 25 per cent had local recurrence only, and 18 per cent had metastases only. At 20 years, 48 per cent of the survivors had metastases and local recurrence. As these figures demonstrate, the adenoid cystic carcinoma tends to run a relentless course. The site of origin has a strong influence on survival (Table 6–2). The site of metastases is most commonly the lungs, followed by bone. Lung metastases do not herald as ominous an outcome with the adenoid cystic carcinoma as they do with other neoplasms. Approximately one-third will be dead within one year. However, 20 per cent will live 5 or more years.[32] On rare occasions, it may even be reasonable to resect a solitary pulmonary metastasis in this disease. This would only be the case if (1) local control seemed assured (this is more likely in the parotid than in other sites) and (2) one were certain that the pulmonary metastasis was solitary. Lymph node involvement is uncommon, occurring in approximately 15 per cent. Even in this small number, it more commonly results from direct extension than from embolic metastasis.[35,36]

The high rate of local recurrence and distant metastases that seems to increase over an indefinite period of time casts a pall over the merits of any proposed treatment plan. There are two classic treatment approaches. Both begin with the premise that the best primary treatment is excision. The first approach advocates complete excision of the tumor, with a partial temporal bone resection if a main branch of the facial nerve is involved. This plan recognizes the tendency of this tumor to travel significant distances along nerves without being grossly apparent. If the tumor recurs, it too is re-

TABLE 6–3   Treatment of Adenoid Cystic Carcinoma

Treatment	5-Year Survival (%)	20-Year Survival (%)
Conservative	82	13
Radical	89	20

sected if possible. This is continued as long as the recurrences are resectable. When a recurrence is unresectable, the patient receives radiation therapy. The second approach is more radical and begins with the largest possible operation that can be devised for the anatomic location.[31] For the parotid, this is a total parotidectomy with sacrifice of the facial nerve and resection of the masseter muscle, ascending ramus of the mandible, and part of the temporal bone in continuity with a radical neck dissection. Recurrences are resected if possible and irradiated if not. The first approach produces 5-year survivals of 82 per cent[5] and 20-year survivals of 13 per cent.[37] The more radical approach produces 5-year survivals of 89 per cent and 20-year survivals of 20 per cent (Table 6–3).

Radiation therapy is used by all for unresectable recurrences. The adenoid cystic carcinoma is said to be radiosensitive, but not radiocurable. Responses are usually good and have been reported to last for as long as 14 years. However the average time from the use of radiation for a recurrence until death in one study was 3.8 years.[38]

A third treatment approach is emerging. This is planned combined therapy. The approach dictates complete excision followed by planned radiation therapy.[39–41] The rationale is that radiation, like resection, works best when the tumor burden is low and that it will never be lower than it is immediately after excision. The number of cases is too small and follow-up too short to know if reality will support the rationale.

MALIGNANT PLEOMORPHIC ADENOMA

At least three different neoplasms are included under the generic term malignant pleomorphic adenoma. Two are malignant from the beginning. One of these is the histologically benign pleomorphic adenoma that metastasizes. This lesion is a clinical and pathologic curiosity.[42,43] The second of these is the tumor with both a malignant epithelial component and a malignant myoepithelial component. Metastases contain both elements. This lesion is then a carcinosarcoma. It too is rare with only a few reported examples.[2]

The third type represents the malignant transformation of the epithelial component within a pre-existing pleomorphic adenoma. Only the epithelial component metastasizes. The preferred terminology for this lesion is the carcinoma ex pleomorphic adenoma coined in 1970.[44] This tumor is unusual, but is being recognized with increasing frequency.[2] The diagnosis can be made if one of the following criteria is met: (1) the presence of a salivary gland malignant neoplasm together with a pleomorphic adenoma, (2) sufficient epithelial anaplasia within a pleomorphic adenoma to classify it as malignant, or (3) destructive or infiltrative growth in a pleomorphic adenoma.[2] The epithelial component is usually a ductal carcinoma.

The carcinoma ex pleomorphic adenoma is variably reported to comprise 0.8 per cent[45] to 9.3 per cent[46] of all salivary gland neoplasms. It accounts for 2 to 5 per cent of the entire pleomorphic adenoma group.[44,47] The sites of origin in decreasing frequency are the parotid, submandibular gland, palate, lip, paranasal sinuses, nasopharynx, and tonsil. This lesion may be easily misdiagnosed on frozen section, with one series reporting an 81 per cent change rate from frozen to permanent sections.[42]

The sex distribution is difficult to determine, with some reporting a strong female predominance[4] and others a strong male predominance.[48] The neoplasm occurs from the second to the ninth decades, but is most common in the fifth to sixth decades. The average age is 10 years older than the pleomorphic adenoma,[2,4] which lends support to the theory of malignant transformation of the epithelial component in a pre-existing pleomorphic adenoma. Further, the classic history is that of long-standing, asymptomatic mass that suddenly manifests rapid growth, often with associated pain. This too supports the theory, as the average duration of the pre-existing mass is 10 years.[42,48] Finally, it has been shown that a portion of the epithelial component of a pleomorphic adenoma develops an increasing DNA content over time.[49]

The carcinoma ex pleomorphic adenoma is more malignant that the more common salivary gland carcinomas. Nodal metastases are present in 25 per cent on initial presentation.[50] Local recurrence after initial resection

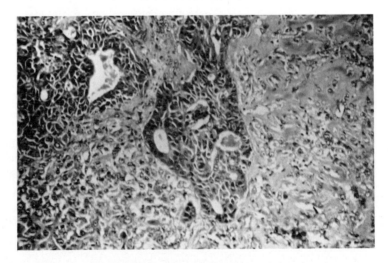

Figure 6–11. Photomicrograph of carcinoma ex pleomorphic adenoma with malignant epithelial component within pleomorphic adenoma.

occurs in 30 per cent.[4] Perineural invasion occurs in up to 50 per cent.[51] Reports of metastases range from 30 per cent[4] to 43 per cent[48] to 70 per cent.[42]

On gross inspection the tumor often appears encapsulated, but may be poorly circumscribed. Necrosis and hemorrhage are common on cut section. Microscopic examination, as already suggested, usually shows vestiges of the pre-existing pleomorphic adenoma (Figure 6–11). Despite the gross appearance of encapsulation, microscopic examination often reveals a breach in the capsule.

The treatment of this lesion is wide excision. For the parotid, this means a total parotidectomy with sacrifice of any portion of the facial nerve near the tumor. Immediate facial nerve repair should be performed. A radical neck dissection should be performed if there is cervical lymphadenopathy, and should be considered even if there is not. Consideration should also be given to postoperative irradiation. Reported 5-year survivals vary from 48 per cent[2] to 62 per cent[5] to 77 per cent.[4] Twenty-year survivals approach zero.

ACINOUS CELL CARCINOMA

According to the Oxford English Dictionary, the proper adjectival form of acinus is acinous. Therefore the correct name for this neoplasm is acinous cell carcinoma. This neoplasm was classified as a benign adenoma until 1953. At that time it was demonstrated that with sufficient follow-up, some behaved in a clearly malignant manner.[52] The majority of investigators now believe that all are malignant, with some being low grade and some high. The high-grade carcinomas manifest intravascular extension, finger-like invasion, and a medullary, ductuloglandular, or primitive tubular growth pattern[2] (to be discussed).

The vast majority occur in the parotid, with the second most common location being the oral cavity, where 62 cases have been reported.[53–55] This tumor represents 2 to 5 per cent all parotid neoplasms and 7 to 19 per cent of all malignant parotid neoplasms. Three per cent are bilateral,[56] a rate of occurrence second only to that of Warthin's tumor. Most cases occur between the ages of 30 and 60 years, but this is second only to the mucoepidermoid carcinoma of salivary gland carcinomas in children.[57] There is a 2 to 1 female prevalence[2] in most reports, but one substantial series[4] reported 76 per cent in males. The acinous cell carcinoma usually appears as a painless, slowly growing mass with an average duration of 6 years.[58]

Gross inspection reveals this neoplasm to be usually unencapsulated, but circumscribed. The cut surface is brittle, gray-white, and solid or

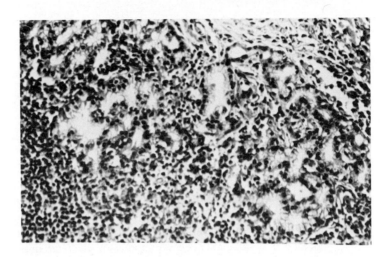

Figure 6–12. Photomicrograph of acinous cell carcinoma of the parotid.

cystic. A variety of patterns have been described microscopically: (1) acinar-lobular, (2) microcystic, (3) follicular, (4) papillary cystic, (5) medullary, (6) ductuloglandular, and (7) primitive tubular. Thirty per cent have a conspicuous lymphoid component, and this tumor, like Warthin's, seems to frequently arise from salivary elements trapped in parotid lymph nodes. Calcification may be prominent (Figure 6–12).

There is considerable disagreement over the proper treatment for this carcinoma because it has been known to recur 1 to 50 years after initial treatment, with an average duration to the time of recurrence of 14 years,[59] and metastases tend to be hematogenous to the lungs and bone, especially the vertebral column. Some favor total parotidectomy with routine radical neck dissection.[60] Others favor excision with clear margins.[61] Some recommend routine resection of the facial nerve,[62] whereas others recommend resection only if the nerve is involved.[63,64]

Recurrences occur in 30 to 50 per cent of cases. Five-year survival figures vary from 47 per cent[5] to 86 per cent[4] to 90 per cent.[60] The 25-year survival is 50 per cent. The average survival before death in one series was 13 years.[62]

A rational treatment approach dictates total parotidectomy as the initial procedure. Any branch of the facial nerve in proximity to the tumor should be resected and immediately repaired. A radical neck dissection need only be performed if there is cervical lymphadenopathy, as the incidence of cervical metastates is 10 per cent.[59,60] Local excision is ill-advised for two reasons: (1) In one study of 69 patients, all who died had only local excision.[64] (2) Radiation seems particularly ineffective for this carcinoma.[65] Recurrences should be treated aggressively with numerous reports attesting to successful salvage.[65] Radiation therapy should be used for unresectable disease, as occasional responses do occur.[55,66]

SQUAMOUS CELL CARCINOMA

Squamous cell carcinomas primary in the salivary glands are unusual. To make the diagnosis one must exclude (1) a high-grade mucoepidermoid carcinoma, (2) metastatic squamous cell carcinoma to the gland or nodes within the gland, (3) invasion of the gland from contiguous structures, and (4) squamous metaplasia within the gland.[67] When this is done, one is left with a small number of tumors (Table 6–4). The true incidence is probably 1 per cent or less of all parotid tumors. This is less than the 1.5 per cent incidence of squamous cell carcinomas of the head and neck that metastasize to the parotid.[69] The incidence is probably similar for the submandibular gland, although an older study reported 12 per cent.[26] Primary squamous cell carcinoma accounts for 3 to 10 per cent of malignant parotid neoplasms.[9,68]

They usually present as firm, indurated masses, and are fixed to surrounding structures in up to 50 per cent.[70] Forty-three per cent extend beyond the confines of the gland,[4] and 25 per cent present with cervical metastases. The tendency to distant metastases has generally been low,[2] although one series recorded an incidence of 25 per cent.[4] A partial or total facial paralysis is noted in 30 per cent. There is a 2 to 1 male prevalence, and the patient is usually over the age of 60 years.

Most authors recommend a total parotidectomy with sacrifice of the facial nerve and immediate repair as the initial treatment. A radical neck dissection should be performed if there is cervical adenopathy, and given serious consideration even if there is not. Most would follow with post-

TABLE 6–4 Primary Squamous Cell Carcinomas of the Parotid Gland

Author	Number of Parotid Tumors	Number of Squamous Cell Carcinomas
Foote and Frazell[26]	766	26 (3.4%)
Batsakis et al.[67]	580	2 (0.3%)
Eneroth[1]	2158	7 (0.3%)
Woods et al.[68]	1360	20 (1.5%)
Spiro et al.[9]	1875	10 (0.5%)
Conley[4]	1538	16 (1.0%)

operative radiation therapy. Five-year survival is approximately 45 per cent.[4,5]

ADENOCARCINOMA

Adenocarcinomas are those primary glandular malignant neoplasms that cannot be classified as adenoid cystic, acinous cell, or mucoepidermoid carcinomas. They account for 2.8 per cent of all parotid neoplasms, and 15 per cent of all parotid carcinomas.[4,71] Several variations have been described, but these are quite unusual. They include the ductal carcinomas[72] and carcinoma of intercalated ducts.[73] Adenocarcinomas on microscopic examination may or may not be papillary, and may or may not be mucus-secreting (Figure 6–13). Invasion of lymphatics and blood vessels is frequent.

They generally are firm-to-hard masses of relatively long duration,[71] and are frequently attached to surrounding structures. They most often occur in the 30- to 60-year age range, and there is probably a slight male predominance. Twenty-two per cent, when first seen, have facial paresis, 25 per cent have regional metastases, and 20 per cent have systemic metastases.[4] As many as 60 per cent evidence spread outside the gland, or, in the parotid, into the deep lobe. Distant metastases are to the skeleton and lungs. Some authors consider them all highly aggressive,[44] whereas others divide them into low and high grades based on histologic invasiveness.[71]

The recommended treatment is wide excision. In the parotid gland

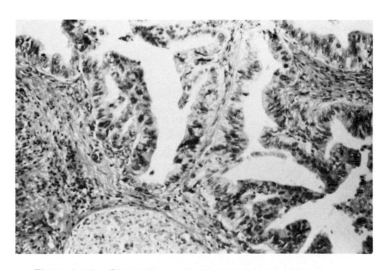

Figure 6–13. Photomicrograph of adenocarcinoma of the parotid.

this means total parotidectomy with sacrifice of the facial nerve with immediate repair. If there is cervical adenopathy, a radical neck dissection should be performed. Many would perform a prophylactic neck dissection. Postoperative irradiation is advised, because the development of a recurrence carries a grave prognosis. Five-year survivals range from 49 per cent[4] to 78 per cent.[71]

UNDIFFERENTIATED CARCINOMA

The undifferentiated carcinomas are those tumors that cannot be classified as adenocarcinomas or squamous cell carcinomas (Figure 6–14) They are uncommon and account for less than 3 per cent of all salivary gland neoplasms, and for 1 to 4.5 per cent of all malignant parotid tumors.[74] They most commonly occur in the seventh to eighth decades, but occur over a wide age range. Approximately one-third appear to arise in a pre-existing pleomorphic adenoma, usually of long duration.[44,75]

Undifferentiated carcinomas are highly malignant. Approximately 33 per cent have partial or total facial paralysis. Forty per cent extend beyond the parotid on presentation.[4] Thirteen per cent present with regional metastases.

The recommended treatment is wide excision. For the parotid, this means total parotidectomy with sacrifice of the facial nerve with immediate repair. Many would include a radical neck dissection. Almost all would

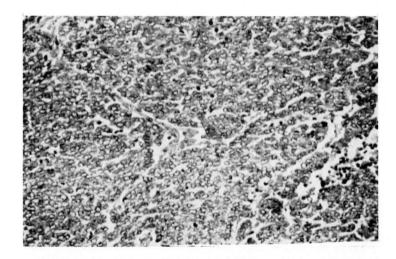

Figure 6–14. Photomicrograph of undifferentiated carcinoma of the parotid.

follow with postoperative irradiation. The 5-year survivals are the lowest of all salivary gland tumors at 25 to 30 per cent.[4,75]

MALIGNANT ONCOCYTOMA

All oncocytomas constitute less than 1 per cent of all salivary gland neoplasms, and the majority are benign. A review in 1977 of the world's literature recorded only 11 cases.[78] On gross inspection the malignant oncocytoma is more apt to be solid than cystic, unlike the benign form. On microscopic examination they may be indistinguishable, although careful review may show evidence of infiltrative, aggressive growth. They are characterized by multiple recurrences and regional metastases, behaving similarly to an adenocarcinoma. Treatment should be planned accordingly.

CLEAR CELL CARCINOMAS

Nonmucinous clear cells within the salivary gland can be classified as glycogen-rich, non-glycogen-containing, and artifactual. The clear cells commonly seen in oncocytomas and acinous cell carcinomas are the result of artifact. There does not exist a clear cell varient of the acinous cell carcinoma.[2,77] The origin of the true clear cell carcinomas is unclear, as all studies have shown them to be relatively undifferentiated, but the myo-

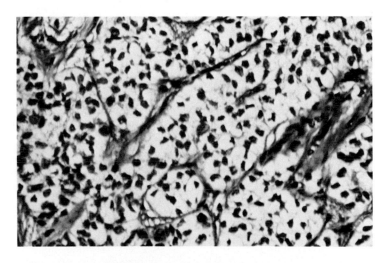

Figure 6–15. Photomicrograph of clear cell carcinoma of the parotid.

epithelial cell is strongly implicated. The cells in the normal salivary gland unit that would correspond most closely are the intercalated duct cell, its corresponding reserve cell, and the myoepithelial cell. Thus, they have also been designated the epithelial-myoepithelial carcinoma of intercalated ducts[73] (Figure 6–15).

These tumors are very rare. Most authorities consider them all to be low-grade carcinomas.[2,73,77,78] Their behavior is akin to that of a low- or intermediate-grade mucoepidermoid carcinoma, and they should be treated accordingly. Finally, they must always be differentiated from metastatic renal cell carcinoma, which may require eliminating the possibility of a renal primary.

NONSALIVARY MALIGNANT NEOPLASMS

Primary fibrosarcomas of the salivary glands are extremely rare. Invasion from contiguous structures must be ruled out. Local recurrence is a hallmark, and wide excision followed by irradiation offers the best chance for cure.

Malignant neurogenous tumors are also rare. They are characterized by local recurrence and a relentless course. In one report of three neurogenous sarcomas and one neuroblastoma,[4] all were treated by radical ablative resection followed by irradiation, and all patients died.

Primary malignant melanoma of the parotid is also rare. The minimum criteria to make this diagnosis are (1) no evidence of a primary melanoma elsewhere, either preoperatively or within 5 years postoperatively, and (2) the presence of melanoma within the substance of the gland and not within a parotid lymph node. The treatment is radical parotidectomy with a radical neck dissection. Consideration should be given to excising the skin over the primary lesion and to including the platysma muscle in the neck dissection specimen so as to include the subdermal lymphatics.

Primary lymphomas of the parotid are rare. The diagnostic criteria include (1) no known extrasalivary lymphoma, (2) histologic proof that the lymphoma involves the salivary gland parenchyma primarily rather than secondarily from the salivary gland node, and (3) architectural and cytologic confirmation of the malignant nature of the lesion. By definition, these lesions are stage I and the prognosis is good.

FACTORS AFFECTING PROGNOSIS

Recent evidence clearly shows that prognosis is more closely related to the stage of the disease than it is to histologic type alone (see the section on general considerations at the beginning of this chapter). Three other factors have been stated to affect the prognosis—facial nerve paralysis, the presence of pain, and the location of the tumor within the parotid.

In one study 46 patients presented with facial paralysis.[79] Seventy-seven per cent of these had metastases. The average length of survival after the onset of paralysis was 2.7 years, and the ultimate mortality was 100 per cent. Another large series[9] reported a 5-year survival of 14 per cent. In a third series,[4] 13 per cent of all patients with malignant neoplasms presented with a partial or total facial paralysis. Sixty per cent of these also had metastases. The 5-year survival was 29 per cent. However, all the survivors had low-grade mucoepidermoid carcinomas, a tumor that only rarely causes facial paralysis. The mortality was 100 per cent within 5 years for all other histologic types. It is clear that pretreatment facial paralysis carries a grave, but not hopeless, prognosis. Treatment should be aggressive. This would mean total parotidectomy, sacrifice of the facial nerve, and possibly partial temporal bone resection. Biopsy of the main trunk of the facial nerve should be obtained at the stylomastoid foramen. If the frozen section examination reveals tumor, a partial temporal bone resection should be performed. Sequential frozen section examinations should be performed until no tumor is seen. Be aware that there may be skip areas, however, especially when dealing with the adenoid cystic carcinoma. A full course of radiation therapy should be given postoperatively.

The presence of pain on initial presentation has also been said to portend an ominous outcome. In one series of 802 parotid neoplasms, pain was present in 5.1 per cent of patients with benign neoplasms and in 6.5 per cent of patients with malignant neoplasms.[7] Thus the presence of pain does not differentiate benign from malignant neoplasms. However, in one series of 288 malignant parotid neoplasms, the 5-year survival rate for those with pain was 35 per cent, whereas for those without pain it was 68 per cent.[9] Similarly, another series found the 5-year survival to be 33 per cent for those with pain and 66 per cent for those without pain.[8] Therefore, if there is pain and if the tumor proves to be malignant, the survival is reduced by approximately 50 per cent.

There is disagreement about whether or not survival is affected by whether the carcinoma is in the deep or superficial lobe. In one large series, location within the deep lobe had a significant adverse effect on prognosis.[4] However, in another large series, the 5-year survival for superficial lobe carcinomas was 69 per cent and for deep lobe tumors was 67 per cent.[9]

METASTATIC DISEASE TO THE PAROTID

There are approximately 20 lymph nodes associated with the parotid gland.[80] They are divided into the paraglandular nodes and the intraglandular nodes, which communicate freely with each other. The paraglandular nodes lie in the subcutaneous layer and are largely pretragal and supratragal in location. They drain the lateral surface of the auricle and the adjacent scalp and cheek. The intraglandular nodes are located within the substance of the gland lateral to the facial vein. Afferent channels drain the nose, eyelids and conjunctiva, the frontotemporal scalp, the external auditory meatus and middle ear, the lacrimal gland, and the sinonasal, nasopharyngeal, and oropharyngeal cavities. Both groups drain to the cervical chain. Because of the location of the paraglandular nodes, metastatic carcinoma must be in the differential diagnosis of any pretragal mass. Because of the location of the intraglandular nodes, lateral to the facial vein where the facial nerve is located, a resection of metastatic disease must also include the facial nerve.

Metastatic carcinoma to the parotid gland is almost always the result of lymphatic embolic spread to the lymph nodes. Contiguous spread and hematogenous spread to the parenchyma are uncommon.[81] High-risk patients are those with deeply invasive melanoma or with poor to moderately differentiated squamous cell carcinoma of the eyelid, conjunctiva, frontotemporal scalp, posterior cheek, or anterior ear. Fifty per cent of these lesions will metastasize at some time in their course, and 33 per cent will have parotid metastases as the first manifestation of metastatic disease.[82]

Melanoma and squamous cell carcinoma account for about 40 per cent each of all metastases to the parotid.[83] Melanoma of the temporal scalp is the single most common offender, and 80 per cent will metastasize to the parotid. Melanoma tends to metastasize to the paraglandular nodes, whereas squamous cell carcinoma tends to spread to the intraglandular nodes.

The majority of these lesions also manifest dissemination to the neck or to distant sites. The latter group is amenable to palliative treatment only, and operative treatment has little place in their therapy. In the absence of distant spread, the treatment plan must be aggressive to offer any hope for cure. The ideal treatment would include excision of the primary in continuity with the parotid gland and a radical neck dissection. The skin from the primary to the parotid should be included as should the platysma muscle in the neck dissection for melanoma. Postoperative irradiation should be given. The usual quoted 5-year survival figures are 12.5 per cent overall, with 11 per cent for melanomas and 14 per cent for squamous cell carcinomas.[4] A recent study reports higher cure rates when routine postoperative irradiation was used, but the follow-up was less than 5 years for some patients.[84]

Infraclavicular primaries with metastases to the parotid are quite rare. In descending order of frequency, the sites are the lungs, breast, kidney, and gastrointestinal tract.

DEEP LOBE PAROTID NEOPLASMS

The deep lobe of the parotid gland is wedged between the ascending ramus of the mandible and the mastoid and tympanic bones. It extends medially toward the pterygomaxillary (parapharyngeal) space anterior to the styloid process, its muscles, and the stylomandibular ligament.

In several large series, deep lobe tumors account for 11 to 12 per cent of all parotid tumors.[86,87] Tumors here may present as a mass below the ear, as a parapharyngeal mass intraorally, or both (the so-called dumbbell tumor). The parapharyngeal presentation is least common.[87] The relative ratio of benign to malignant is the same as for the superficial lobe, with approximately 20 to 25 per cent being malignant.[86] Mucoepidermoid and acinous cell carcinomas are the most common. There is considerable disparity in reported cure rates. (See the section on Factors Affecting Prognosis in this chapter.) Wide excision is mandatory for these malignant tumors, but this need not necessitate sacrifice of the facial nerve, which may be a safe distance from the tumor.[85] Nineteen per cent manifest cervical metastases, and consideration should be given to a radical neck dissection for high-grade tumors. Since the resection margins would almost certainly be close, postoperative irradiation should be used even for low-grade malignant neoplasms.

SUBMANDIBULAR, SUBLINGUAL, AND MINOR SALIVARY GLAND CARCINOMAS

Fifty per cent of submandibular gland tumors are malignant. They are of the same histologic type as occur in the parotid, but in general are more aggressive. The relative frequency is also different. In two large series, the relative frequencies were: (1) adenoid cystic carcinoma, 30 per cent; mucoepidermoid carcinoma, 30 per cent; and adenocarcinoma, 16 per cent;[4] and (2) adenoid cystic carcinoma, 30 per cent; adenocarcinoma, 30 per cent; and undifferentiated carcinoma, 30 per cent.[88] Five-year survivals are poor, being approximately 10 per cent for adenoid cystic carcinomas, 17 per cent for mucoepidermoid carcinomas, and 0 per cent for adenocarcinomas. Contemporary thinking favors a composite resection.[89] Many would include a radical neck dissection, and postoperative irradiation is strongly recommended.[90]

Tumors of the sublingual gland are unusual. Eighty per cent are malignant, with the adenoid cystic carcinoma and the mucoepidermoid carcinoma accounting for 40 per cent each. The presenting symptom is always a submucosal mass under the anterior tongue. Treatment and survival figures are similar to those for the submandibular gland.

Minor salivary gland tumors are equal to or more frequent than tumors of the submandibular gland. Fifty to 65 per cent are malignant. The majority occur in the oral cavity, with 50 per cent of those on the palate. Most present as a mass only, although 18 per cent also are painful, and these are always adenoid cystic carcinomas. In all locations, the adenoid cystic carcinoma predominates and accounts for 35 to 40 per cent of all malignant tumors. It is more aggressive in the minor glands than in the parotid. Fourteen per cent[32] to 16 per cent[91] demonstrate lymph node metastases. Distant metastases occur in 40 per cent, usually to lungs, bone, and brain in descending frequency. The preferred treatment is the widest possible excision.[31] Strong consideration should be given to postoperative irradiation, as the overall 5-year survival with excision alone as primary therapy is 8 per cent.[4]

Second in frequency in most series is the adenocarcinoma, and third is the mucoepidermoid carcinoma. These are also marked by aggressive behavior, with regional metastases in 31 per cent and distant metastases in up to 51 per cent. Again wide excision is the recommended treatment, with consideration of postoperative irradiation. The overall 5-year survivals reported are usually around 44 per cent; at 10 years it is 32 per cent.[92]

Minor salivary gland carcinomas account for 4 to 8 per cent of all malignant neoplasms of the nose and paranasal sinuses. In descending order of frequency, they are the adenoid cystic carcinoma, the adenocarcinoma, the mucoepidermoid carcinoma, and the undifferentiated carcinoma. It has been known for over a decade that there is an increased incidence of adenocarcinoma in workers in the furniture and footwear industries.[93–96] The recommended treatment, when possible, is wide excision followed by planned irradiation. Postoperative radiation therapy is preferred because this reduces the chance of geographic miss.[97] If the lesion is unresectable, radiation alone is given. The overall 5-year survival is 15 per cent.[92]

Forty per cent of all minor salivary gland tumors of the oral cavity are malignant.[98] The most common locations are the palate and the tongue. The adenoid cystic carcinoma is most frequent followed by the mucoepidermoid carcinoma, and the adenocarcinoma. The best treatment is wide excision with postoperative irradiation.[99] The 5-year survival for low-grade mucoepidermoid carcinomas is 100 per cent; for high-grade tumors it is 17 per cent. The 5-year survival for the adenoid cystic carcinoma and the adenocarcinoma is 10 to 20 per cent.[100] As has been stated, however, the adenoid cystic carcinoma ''may give a respectable 3-year survival, but the survival drops sharply at 5 years and is disastrous at 6 to 8 years.''[101]

Minor salivary gland carcinomas account for less than 1 per cent of all carcinomas of the larynx.[102,103] In descending order of frequency they are the adenoid cystic carcinoma, the adenocarcinoma, the mucoepidermoid carcinoma, and the very rare carcinoma ex pleomorphic adenoma. Supraglottic and subglottic lesions occur with equal frequency. The peak incidence is in the fifth to sixth decade. Twenty-seven per cent present with cervical metastases. An aggressive treatment plan should be followed, as the survival figures are poor. Treatment should include a total laryngectomy with a radical neck dissection for cervical adenopathy. Consideration should be given to a prophylactic neck dissection if the lesion is clearly unilateral. Postoperative irradiation should be employed. Five-year survivals are 12 per cent for the adenoid cystic carcinoma and 28 per cent for the adenocarcinoma, with the majority of the latter dying within 2 years.[104]

Tracheal carcinomas are rare. The adenoid cystic carcinoma accounts for 20 to 25 per cent of all tracheal malignant neoplasms and is twice as common as the adenocarcinoma. These tumors have a predilection for the upper third of the trachea, and this is fortunate because the survivals are better the more cephalic the lesion. Sixty per cent occur on the posterior or lateral walls. The best treatment, when possible, is resection with end-to-end anastomosis combined with a paratracheal and upper mediastinal node dissection.[105] It has been stated that irradiation should not be used as it may lead to a tracheomediastinal fistula.[106] The 3-year survival is 13 per cent.

On rare occasions malignant salivary gland tumors can arise in aberrant salivary tissue as discussed in the chapter on Benign Neoplasms. The most common is the mucoepidermoid carcinoma, followed by the adenoid cystic carcinoma.

MALIGNANT NEOPLASMS IN CHILDREN

Salivary gland tumors in children are rare and constitute less than 5 per cent of all salivary gland neoplasms.[107,108] Twenty-five to 35 per cent of these are malignant.[109] The mucoepidermoid carcinoma is most common, followed by the acinous cell carcinoma. There is no evidence to suggest a different biologic course from that observed in adults. Therefore the treatment should be the same. Irradiation in children carries a significant long-term risk and should be used with discretion.

CONTROVERSIAL TREATMENT MODALITIES

Radical Neck Dissection

There is considerable disagreement in the literature about the role of the radical neck dissection in the management of salivary gland carcinomas. All agree that a radical neck dissection should be performed for palpable cervical adenopathy. The disagreement is over the prophylactic neck dissection. In one large series, radical neck dissection was performed in only 15 per cent of patients with parotid carcinomas.[110] In another large series it was noted that in the absence of recurrence at the primary site, only 5 per cent of patients developed regional or distant metastases.[92] Others take a more aggressive stance and recommend prophylactic neck dissection for a significant percentage of cases, especially squamous cell carcinomas and high-grade mucoepidermoid carcinomas.[4]

The weight of the world's literature would support the position of not doing a prophylactic neck dissection for the majority of parotid carcinomas. For T3 lesions, a prophylactic neck dissection would seem reasonable for the high-grade carcinomas that tend to develop lymphatic metastases. These are the high-grade adenocarcinomas and mucoepidermoid carcinomas, squamous cell carcinomas, and carcinomas ex pleomorphic adenoma. A similar policy would seem rational for the submandibular and sublingual glands. Since carcinomas in these 2 sites have a reduced survival, care must be taken to get an adequate block resection around the tumor. Simple excision of the gland is inadequate.

A different approach seems necessary for the minor glands. Apparently a prophylactic neck dissection is never indicated for those lesions arising superior to a horizontal plane from the oral commissure to the lobule. In this situation, excision of the primary and the radical neck dissection would always theoretically leave tumor between the two sites. For lesions in the tongue and floor of the mouth an in-continuity dissection could be performed, but statistically would only seem reasonable for the very large lesions.

Irradiation

The use of irradiation in the treatment of salivary carcinomas continues to be expanded. At one time irradiation was believed to be relatively ineffective and was reserved for inoperable disease. This policy clearly placed the modality at a distinct disadvantage. Irradiation, like excision, works best when facing a small tumor burden. In recent years more and more studies have shown irradiation to be efficacious when the tumor burden is small.

One study reported a reduction in local recurrence from 36 to 11 percent with the use of routine postoperative radiation for high-grade carcinomas.[111] One review of 93 salivary carcinomas found that conservative excision followed by irradiation produced equal survival figures to radical excision alone.[112] Another reported a higher 5-year survival with conservative resection followed by irradiation than that achieved with radical resection alone.[113] One remarkable study reported a 49.7 per cent 5-year survival for patients with facial nerve paralysis with combined excision and postoperative irradiation.[114] This is far superior to any other report on patients with facial nerve paralysis.[9-11] Irradiation may get even better. A recent report recorded 100 per cent local control with fast neutron therapy versus 33 per cent local control with cobalt therapy for large carcinomas.[115] There is still general agreement that the acinous cell carcinoma is uniquely unresponsive to irradiation.[65]

At this time the indications for irradiation would seem to be (1) for known or suspected residual disease, (2) for all high-grade carcinomas, (3) for unresectable carcinomas, and (4) for all carcinomas of the deep lobe.

REFERENCES

1. Eneroth CM: Salivary gland tumors in the parotid gland, submandibular gland, and the palate region. Cancer 27:1415, 1971.
2. Batsakis JG: *Tumors of the Head and Neck.* Williams & Wilkins, Baltimore, 1979.
3. Ackerman LV, del Regato JA: *Cancer - Diagnosis, Treatment and Prognosis.* 3rd Ed, C. V. Mosby Company, St. Louis, 1962.
4. Conley J: *Salivary Glands and the Facial Nerve.* Grune and Stratton, New York, 1975.
5. Johns ME, Coulthard SW: Survival and follow-up in malignant tumors of the salivary glands. Otolaryngol Clin N Amer 10:455, 1977.
6. Clark SK, Yarington CT Jr: Lingual malignant disease of minor salivary gland origin. Am J Otolaryngol 1:181, 1980.
7. Eneroth CM: Histological and clinical aspects of parotid tumors. Acta Otolaryngol (Suppl 191) 1963.
8. Mustard RA, Anderson W: Malignant tumors of the parotid gland. Ann Surg 159:291, 1964.
9. Spiro RH, Huvos AF, Strong EW: Cancer of the parotid gland. A clinicopathologic study of 288 primary cases. Am J Surg 130:452, 1975.
10. Eneroth CM, Hamberger CA: Principles of treatment of different types of parotid tumors. Laryngoscope 84:1732, 1974.
11. Conley J, Hamaker RC: Prognosis of malignant tumors of the parotid gland with facial paralysis. Arch Otolaryngol 101:39, 1975.
12. Kagan AR, Nussbaum H, Handler S, Shapiro R, Gilbert HA, Jacobs M, Miles JW, Chan PYM, Calcaterra T: Recurrences from malignant parotid gland tumors. Cancer 37:2600, 1976.
13. Rice DH, Batsakis JG, McClatchey KD: Postirradiation malignant salivary gland tumor. Arch Otolaryngol 102:699, 1976.
14. Berg JW, Hutter RVP, Foote FW Jr: The unique association between salivary gland cancer and breast cancer. JAMA 204:771, 1968.
15. Prior P, Waterhouse JAH: Second primary cancer in patients with tumors of the salivary glands. Br J Cancer 36:362, 1977.
16. Levitt SH, McHugh RB, Gomez-Marin O, Hyams VJ, Soule EH, Strong EW, Sellers AH, Woods JE, Guillamondegui OM: Clinical staging system for cancer of the salivary gland: a retrospective study. Cancer 47:2712, 1981.
17. Cited in Thorvaldsson SE, Beahrs OH, Woolner LB, Simons JN: Mucoepidermoid tumors of the major salivary glands. Am J Surg 120:432, 1970.
18. Stewart FW, Foote FW Jr, Becker WF: Mucoepidermoid tumors of the salivary glands. Am Surg 122:820, 1945.
19. Frazell EL: Clinical aspects of tumors of the major salivary glands. Cancer 7:637, 1954.

20. Jakobsson PA, Blanck C, Eneroth CM: Mucoepidermoid carcinoma of the parotid gland. Cancer 22:111, 1968.
21. Stevenson DF, Hazard JF: Mucoepidermoid carcinoma of salivary gland origin. Cleve Clin Q 20:445, 1953.
22. Eneroth CM, Zetterberg A: The relationship between the nuclear DNA content in smears of aspirates and prognosis of mucoepidermoid carcinoma. Acta Otolaryngol 80:429, 1975.
23. Eneroth CM, Zetterberg A: A cytochemical method of grading the malignancy of salivary gland tumors preoperatively. Acta Otolaryngol 81:489, 1976.
24. Thorvaldson SE, Beahrs OH, Woolner LB, Simons JN: Mucoepidermoid tumors of the major salivary glands. AM J Surg 120:432, 1970.
25. Eneroth CM, Hjertman L, Moberger G: Mucoepidermoid carcinoma of the palate. Acta Otolaryngol 70:408, 1970.
26. Foote FW Jr, Frazell EL: Tumors of the major salivary glands. Cancer 6:1065, 1953.
27. Billroth T: Beobachtungen uber Geschwulste der Speicheldrusen. Virchow's Arch (Pathol Anat) 17:357, 1857.
28. Leefstedt SW, Gaeta JF, Sako K, Marchetta FC, Shedd DP: Adenoid cystic carcinoma of major and minor salivary glands. Am J Surg 122:756, 1971.
29. Berdal R, de Besche A, Mylius E: Cylindroma of salivary glands: Report of 80 cases. Acta Otolaryngol 263:170, 1970.
30. Ballantyne AJ, McCarter AB, Ibanez ML: The extension of cancer of the head and neck through peripheral nerves. Am J Surg 106:651, 1963.
31. Conley J, Dingman DL: Adenoid cystic carcinoma of the head and neck (cylindroma). Arch Otolaryngol 100:81, 1974.
32. Spiro RH, Huvos AG, Strong EW: Adenoid cystic carcinoma of salivary origin. A clinicopathologic study of 242 cases. Am J Surg 128:512, 1974.
33. Fu KK, Leibel SA, Levine ML, Friedlander LM, Boles R, Philips TL: Carcinoma of the major and minor salivary glands. Analysis of treatment results and sites and causes of failures. Cancer 40:2882, 1977.
34. Osborn DA: Morphology and the natural history of cribriform adenocarcinoma (adenoid cystic carcinoma). J Clin Pathol 30:195, 1977.
35. Ganzer U: Behandlung und prognose des adenoidzystischen karzinoms. Laryngol Rhinol 53:901, 1974.
36. Allen MS Jr, Marsh WL Jr: Lymph node involvement by direct extension in adenoid cystic carcinoma. Absence of classic embolic lymph node metastasis. Cancer 38:2017, 1976.
37. Blanck C, Eneroth CM, Jacobsson PA: Adenoid cystic carcinoma of the parotid gland. Acta Radiol Scand 6:177, 1967.
38. Seaver PR Jr, Kuehn PG: Adenoid cystic carcinoma of the salivary glands. Am J Surg 137:449, 1979.
39. Rich DH: Adenoid cystic carcinoma of the minor salivary glands: long-term survival with planned combined therapy. Arch Otolaryngol 107:128, 1981.
40. Black KM, Fitzpatrick PH, Palmer JA: Adenoid cystic carcinoma of the salivary glands. Can J Surg 23:32, 1980.
41. Gleave EN, Whittaker JS, Nicholson A: Salivary tumors—experience over thirty years. Clin Otolaryngol 4:247, 1979.
42. Gerughty RM, Scofield HH, Brown FM, Hennigar GR: Malignant mixed tumors of salivary gland origin. Cancer 24:471, 1969.
43. Youngs GR, Scheuer PJ: Histologically benign mixed parotid tumour with hepatic metastasis. J Pathol 109:171, 1973.
44. Evans RW, Cruickshank AH: *Epithelial Tumors of the Salivary Glands*, W. B. Saunders, Philadelphia, 1970.
45. Freeman FM, Beahrs OH, Wollner LB: Surgical treatment of malignant tumors of the parotid gland. Am J Surg 110:527, 1965.
46. Morgan MN, Mackenzie OH: Tumours of salivary glands: a review of 204 cases with five years follow-up. Br J Surg 55:284, 1968.

47. Beahrs OH, Woolner LB, Kirklin JW, Devine KD: Carcinomatous transformation of mixed tumors of the parotid gland. Arch Surg 75:605, 1957.
48. Eneroth CM, Blanck D, Jakobsson PA: Carcinoma in pleomorphic adenoma of the parotid gland. Acta Otolaryngol 66:477, 1968.
49 Eneroth CM, Zetterberg A: Malignancy in pleomorphic adenoma. A clinical and microspectrophotometric study. Acta Otolaryngol 77:426, 1974.
50. Spiro RH, Huvos AG, Strong EW: Malignant mixed tumor of salivary origin. A clinicopathologic study of 146 cases. Cancer 38:388, 1977.
51. LiVolsi VA, Perzin KH: Malignant mixed tumors arising in salivary glands. I. Carcinomas arising in benign mixed tumors: a clinicopathologic study. Cancer 39:2209, 1977.
52. Buxton RW, Maxwell JH, French AJ: Surgical treatment of epithelial tumors of the parotid gland. Surg Gynecol Obstet 97:401, 1953.
53. Gardner DG, Bell ME, Wesley RK, Wysochi GP: Acinic cell tumors of minor salivary glands. Oral Surg 50:545, 1980.
54. Ferlito A: Acinic cell carcinoma of minor salivary glands. Histopathology 4:331, 1980.
55. Hutchinson JC Jr: Acinic cell carcinoma of minor salivary gland origin. Am J Otolaryngol 2:54, 1981.
56. Levin JM, Robinson DW, Lin F: Acinic cell carcinoma: collective review, including bilateral cases. Arch Surg 110:64, 1975.
57. Krolls SO, Trodahl JN, Boyers RC: Salivary gland lesions in children: a survey of 430 cases. Cancer 30:459, 1972.
58. Abrams AM, Cornyn J, Scofield HH, Hansen LSL: Acinic cell adenocarcinoma of the major salivary glands: Clinicopathologic study of 77 cases. Cancer 18:1145, 1965.
59. Fox NM Jr, ReMine WII, Woolner LB: Acinic cell carcinoma of the major salivary glands. Am J Surg 106, 860, 1963.
60. Eneroth CM, Hamberger CA, Jakobsson PA: Malignancy of acinic cell carcinoma. Ann Otol Rhinol Laryngol 75:780, 1966.
61. Godwin JT, Foote FW, Frazell EL: Acinic cell adenocarcinoma of the parotid gland. Am J Pathol 30:465, 1954.
62. Grage TB, Lober PH, Arhelger SW: Acinic cell carcinoma of the parotid gland. Am J Surg 102:765, 1961.
63. Spiro RH, Huvos AG, Strong EW: Acinic cell carcinoma of salivary origin. A clinicopathologic study of 67 cases. Cancer 41:924, 1978.
64. Chong GC, Beahrs OH, Wollner LB: Surgical management of acinic cell carcinoma of the parotid gland. Surg Gynec Obstet 138:65, 1974.
65. Perzin KH, LiVolsi VA: Acinic cell carcinomas arising in salivary glands: a clinicopathologic study. Cancer 44:1434, 1979.
66. Fermont DC: Acinic cell carcinoma of intraoral minor salivary gland origin. J. Laryngol Otol 93:423, 1979.
67. Batsakis JG, McClatchey KD, Johns ME, Regazi J: Primary squamous cell carcinoma of the parotid gland. Arch Otolaryngol 102:355, 1976.
68. Woods JE, Chong GC, Beahrs OH: Experience with 1360 primary parotid tumors. Ann J Surg 130:460, 1975.
69 Ridenhour CE, Pratt JS Jr: Epidermoid carcinoma of the skin involving the parotid gland. Am J Surg 112:504, 1966.
70. Epker BN: Clinical and histopathological aspects of salivary gland tumors. Henry Ford Hosp Med J 15:345, 1967.
71. Blanck C, Eneroth CM, Jacobsson PA: Mucous-producing adenopapillary (non-epidermoid) carcinoma of the parotid gland. Cancer 28:676, 1971.
72. Gaisford JC, Hanna DC, Sotereanos GC: Primary cancer of Stenson's duct. Arch Otolaryngol 82:45, 1965.
73. Corio RL, Sciubba JJ, Brennon RB, Batsakis JG: Epithelial-myoepithelial carcinoma of intercalated duct origin. Oral Surg Oral Med Oral Pathol 53:280, 1982.
74. Blanck C, Backstrom A, Eneroth CM, Jakobsson PA: Poorly differentiated solid parotid carcinoma. Acta Radiol 13:17, 1974.

75. Patey DH, Thackray AC, Keeling DH: Malignant disease of the parotid. Br J Cancer 19:712, 1965.
76. Johns ME, Regezi JA, Batsakis JG: Oncocytic neoplasms of salivary glands: an ultrastructural study. Laryngoscope 87:862, 1977.
77. Echevarria RA: Ultrastructure of the acinic cell carcinoma and clear cell carcinoma of the parotid gland. Cancer 20:563, 1967.
78. Mohamed AH, Cherrick HM: Glycogen-rich adenocarcinoma of minor salivary glands: a light and electron microscopic study. Cancer 36:1057, 1975.
79. Eneroth CM: Facial nerve paralysis. Arch Otolaryngol 95:300, 1972.
80. Haagensen CR, Feinal CR, Herter FP, Slanety CA, Weinberg JA: *The Lymphatics in Cancer.* W. B. Saunders Company, Philadelphia, 1972, pp. 63–71.
81. Conley J, Arena S: Parotid gland as a focus of metastasis. Arch Surg 87:757, 1963.
82. Storm FK, Eilber FR, Sparks FC, Morton DL: A prospective study of parotid metastases from head and neck cancer. Am J Surg 134:115, 1977.
83. Pope TH Jr, Lehmann WB: Parotid metastasis to parotid nodes. Arch Otolaryngol 86:673, 1967.
84. Rees R, Maples M, Lynch JA, Rosenfeld L: Malignant secondary parotid tumors. South Med J 74:1050, 1981.
85. Nigro MF, Spiro RH: Deep lobe parotid tumors. Am J Surg 134:523, 1977.
86. Hanna DC, Gaisford JC, Richardson GS, Bindra RN: Tumors of the deep lobe of the parotid gland. Am J Surg 116:524, 1968.
87. Eneroth CM: Discussion of paper by Berdal P, Gronas HE, Mylius EA: Parotid tumors: clinical and histological aspects. Acta Otolaryngol 263:160, 1970.
88. Rafla S: Submaxillary gland tumors. Cancer 26:821, 1970.
89. Spiro RH, Hajdu SI, Strong EW: Tumors of the submaxillary gland. Am J Surg 132:463, 1976.
90. Hanna DC, Clairmont AA: Submandibular gland tumors. Plast Reconstr Surg 61:198, 1978.
91. Osborn DA: Morphology and the natural history of cribriform adenocarcinomas (adenoid cystic carcinoma). J Clin Pathol 30:195, 1977.
92. Spiro RH, Koss LG, Hajdu SI, Strong EW: Tumors of minor salivary origin: a clinicopathologic study of 492 cases. Cancer 31:117, 1973.
93. Hadfield ES: A study of adenocarcinomas of the paranasal sinuses in woodworkers in the furniture industry. Ann R Coll Surg Engl 46:301, 1969.
94. Acheson ED, Cowdell RH, Rang E: Adenocarcinoma of the nasal cavity and sinuses in England and Wales. Br J Ind Med 29:21, 1972.
95. MacBeth R: Malignant disease of the paranasal sinuses. J Laryngol 79:593, 1965.
96. Brinton LA, Blot WJ, Stone BJ, Braumeni JF Jr: A death certificate analysis of nasal cancer among furniture workers in North Carolina. Can Res 37:3473, 1977.
97. Boone ML, Harle TS, Highholt HW, Fletcher GH: Malignant disease of the paranasal sinuses and nasal cavity. Am J Roentgenol 102:627, 1968.
98. Chaudry AP, Vickers RA, Gorlin RJ: Intraoral minor salivary gland tumors. Oral Surg 14:1194, 1961.
99. Gregor RT, Heng BB: Minor salivary gland carcinomas of the mouth and orapharynx. J Otolaryngol 10:267, 1981.
100. Adams DL, Duvall AJ: Adenocarcinoma of the head and neck. Arch Otolaryngol 93:261, 1971.
101. Shumrick DA: Treatment of malignant tumors of minor salivary glands. Arch Otolaryngol 88:74, 1968.
102. Houle JA, Joseph P, Batsakis JG: Primary adenocarcinoma of the larynx. J Laryngol 90:1159, 1976.
103. Olofsson J, Van Nostrand AWP: Adenoid cystic carcinoma of the larynx. A report of four cases and a review of literature. Cancer 40:1307, 1977.
104. Fechner RE: Adenocracinoma of the larynx. Canad J Otolaryngol 4:284, 1975.
105. McCafferty GJ, Parker LS, Suggit SC: Primary malignant disease of the trachea. J Laryngol Otol 78:331, 1964.

106. Birt BD: The management of malignant tracheal neoplasms. J Laryngol Otol 84:723, 1970.
107. Castro EB, Huvos AG, Strong EW, Foote FW Jr: Tumors of the major salivary glands in children. Cancer 29:312, 1972.
108. Kauffman SL, Stout AP: Tumors of the major salivary glands in children. Cancer 16:1317, 1963.
109. Schuller DE, McCabe BF: The firm salivary mass in children. Laryngoscope 87:189, 1977.
110. Woods JE, Weiland LH, Chong GC, Irons GB: Pathology and surgery of primary tumors of the parotid. Surg Clin North Am 57:565, 1977.
111. Fletcher GH, Jesse RH: The place of irradiation in the management of the primary lesion in head and neck cancers. Cancer 39:862, 1977.
112. Boles R, Raines J, Lebovits M, Fu KK: Malignant tumors of salivary glands: a university experience. Laryngoscope 90:729, 1980.
113. Reinfuss M, Korzeniowski S: The role of radiotherapy in the treatment of malignant tumors of the salivary glands. Tumori 66:467, 1980.
114. Byun YS, Fayos JV, Kim YH: Management of malignant salivary gland tumors. Laryngoscope 90:1052, 1980.
115. Henry LW, Blasko JC, Griffin TW, Parker RG: Evaluation of fast neutron teletherapy for advanced carcinomas of the major salivary glands. Cancer 44:814, 1979.

INDEX

149